Success Stories

"It is so wonderful to find another doctor who cares about really helping people. You have done much more for my son and me than many other doctors I have seen face to face. I rank you with Dr. Cannell, Dr. Heaney, Dr. Mercola, and Dr. Jonathan Wright." —**Twyla Holstein**

"Your book is the first that speaks directly to me. I have started following the detox plan and feel confident that I am safely taking the steps to feel the best I can.

This is the first literature that I have found that clearly addresses the autoimmune component of Hashimoto's and provides straightforward information and tools to empower me to take charge of my well-being. Thanks so much for your information and knowledge!" —**Libby Dixon**

"I started The Hypothyroid diet six days ago and I have lost 4.6 lbs. I will say that I truly feel good for a change. It has been a while since I have felt good. I would recommend this diet to ALL the people that have hypothyroidism." —**Mari Steele**

"I can't stop reading this book. I couldn't believe how bad certain foods were for hypothyroidism. I felt so much better after two days it was unbelievable! My mind feels alert and my body feels lighter. Thank you for coming into my life with your books." —**Jean Gear**

THE HypoThyroid DIET

Lose Weight and Beat Fatigue in 21 Days

Kevin Dobrzynski, D.N.

New York

THE HypoThyroid DIET
Lose Weight and Beat Fatigue in 21 Days

Kevin Dobrzynski, D.N.

Disclaimer: The Publisher and the Author make no representations or warranties with respect to the accuracy or completeness of the contents of this work and specifically disclaim all warranties, including without limitation warranties of fitness for a particular purpose. No warranty may be created or extended by sales or promotional materials. The advice and strategies contained herein may not be suitable for every situation. This work is sold with the understanding that the Publisher is not engaged in rendering legal, accounting, or other professional services. If professional assistance is required, the services of a competent professional person should be sought. Neither the Publisher nor the Author shall be liable for damages arising herefrom. The fact that an organization or website is referred to in this work as a citation and/or a potential source of further information does not mean that the Author or the Publisher endorses the information the organization or website may provide or recommendations it may make. Further, readers should be aware that internet websites listed in this work may have changed or disappeared between when this work was written and when it is read.

The information and recommendations outlined in this book are not intended as a substitute of personalized medical advice; the reader of this book should see a qualified health care provider. This book proposes certain theoretical methods of nutrition not necessarily mainstream.

It is left to the discretion and it is the sole responsibility of the user of the information indicated in this book to determine if procedures and recommendations described are appropriate. The author of this information cannot be held responsible for the information or any inadvertent errors or omissions of the information.

The information in this presentation should not be construed as a claim or representation that any procedure or product mentioned constitutes a specific cure, palliative, or ameliorative. Procedures and nutritional compounds described should be considered as adjunctive to other accepted conventional procedures deemed necessary by the attending licensed doctor. It is the concern of the Department of Health and Human Services that no homeopathic or nutritional supplements be used to replace established, conventional medical approaches, especially in cases of emergencies, serious or life-threatening diseases, or conditions.

I share in this concern, as replacing conventional treatment with such remedies, especially in serious cases, may deprive the patient of necessary treatment and thereby cause harm as well as potentially pose a major legal liability for the health professional involved. The nutritional compounds mentioned in this book should not be used as replacements for conventional medical treatment.

The Food and Drug Administration has not evaluated the information detailed in this document. The nutritional supplements mentioned in this manual are not intended to diagnose, treat, cure, or prevent disease.

ISBN 978-1-61448-030-3 Paperback
ISBN 978-1-61448-147-8 eBook
Library of Congress Control Number: 2011942399

Published by:

MORGAN JAMES PUBLISHING
The Entrepreneurial Publisher
5 Penn Plaza, 23rd Floor
New York City, New York 10001
(212) 655-5470 Office
(516) 908-4496 Fax
www.MorganJamesPublishing.com

Cover Design by:
Rachel Lopez
rachel@r2cdesign.com

Interior Design by:
Bonnie Bushman
bbushman@bresnan.net

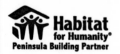

Habitat for Humanity
Peninsula Building Partner

In an effort to support local communities, raise awareness and funds, Morgan James Publishing donates a percent of all book sales for the life of each book to Habitat for Humanity Peninsula and Greater Williamsburg.
Get involved today, visit
www.HelpHabitatForHumanity.org.

Dedication

This book is dedicated to my wife Amy, without your struggle this book would have not been possible. For Brook and Dean, it's for you that I do what I do. And to the millions who suffer from hypothyroidism, let this be the starting point to your recovery.

To my parents who gave me the support and foundation for a future filled with opportunity.

Foreword

This book is not intended to diagnose, treat or cure hypothyroidism. Instead, this program is designed to boost your immune system, reduce stress on the many systems of the human body, and help you lose weight.

Stress comes in many forms...chemical, physical, mental, emotional, internal and/or external.

When your body is free from stress, it can heal itself from most ailments and/or diseases that infect it, assuming it's given the right nourishment.

Reducing stress will raise your metabolic rate, making your body much more efficient at losing and maintaining normal body weight.

This book will cover the biochemical stress placed on your body through all substances you feed it directly or indirectly and lay out a simple step-by-step plan on how to reduce the biochemical stress.

It will show you what foods can place a burden on the body through food sensitivities. These reactions will make it harder for you to lose weight.

There will also be a section on how to nourish and support your thyroid and other organs that communicate with the thyroid.

To get the most out of the book, don't treat it like another diet book. Approach this book like a step-by-step program prescribed by a physician, because this is exactly what it is.

There will be a few recommendations in this book in regards to supplementation. However, following the food plan will have a bigger impact on how much weight you lose and how you feel compared to any supplement or combination of supplements you take.

There is nothing that impacts the body more than the food you eat and what you drink six to ten times per day.

You may notice that there are no references in this book. This is not because what is being described here is fictitious.

The information compiled in this book is from years of experience working with patients who have weight issues, hypothyroidism, and other chronic conditions, along with information gained from other medical authorities in natural and traditional medicine.

The information in this book works if you use it with consistency and conviction.

Remember one thing, there will not be one action, food, or drug that will make you feel better overnight or help you lose 20 pounds in a week.

It's the consistent use of nutritious food and drink and the elimination of toxic substances that will support the body so it can heal and rid itself of excess weight.

One important thing you can do when eating/drinking is to pay attention to what your body is trying to tell you and whether or not your body agrees with what you ate.

For example, after ingesting a meal, do you have the tendency to burp or belch in excess?

This may be a sign/symptom that your body doesn't like what you've just consumed or the combination of foods you ate is causing the problem.

Your body is an amazing machine, and it will tell you what it likes or dislikes—you just have to listen. I will tell you how to do this.

There will be information on how to combine foods to make it easier on your body to digest.

There will be information on how to design the perfect meal for you and no one else just by paying attention to how you feel after a meal.

There will be information on how to eliminate food cravings, sensitivities, and allergies.

And last but not least, there will be information on how to increase your metabolism so that your body can burn fat around the clock.

This is not a plan to try out for two or three weeks so you can lose a few pounds.

This program is designed to be followed for life. If you follow this plan as a routine way of eating daily, I ensure you'll have many long years without weight problems and chronic health conditions.

This book was written as a lifestyle guide for you—the hypothyroid patient so that you can lose weight and feel normal again.

There is a lot of confusion about what to eat and what not to eat when you have hypothyroidism. This book provides a blueprint to follow without the confusion.

The inspiration for this book is my wife who suffers from hypothyroidism even though she is being treated with prescription medication for her condition.

In fact, she has no thyroid...it was removed in February 2010 due to extremely large nodules.

The bad news was her thyroid contained malignant cells, the good news is—they've been removed.

My wife is a testament that you can feel better and live a normal life and look great if you follow the right diet.

This book is also for the many millions of people who are diagnosed annually with hypothyroidism, yet still suffer from the condition because of a failing medical system.

Remember, you are not just a number; you are not your disease unless you give into the disease.

Fight back by following this guide, don't give in until you feel better and you're in control of your health.

When you have your health—true health, you'll have no problems with your weight.

Dr. Kevin Dobrzynski DN

Table of Contents

Introduction

You're already aware that you have hypothyroidism; you're familiar with the symptoms, and you may even know how your thyroid works.

What you may not know is how diet plays a crucial role in feeling better and losing weight with hypothyroidism.

Hopefully, your doctor has done a good job at diagnosing and medicating your condition. This will keep your blood test results within the *normal* range of someone with no thyroid problem.

However, there's a good chance you may still be dealing with symptoms from this condition.

This is because a majority of hypothyroid patients have Hashimoto's thyroiditis—which is an autoimmune disorder.

The problem is not that your thyroid is broken, but that your immune system is not functioning correctly and it's inadvertently attacking your thyroid.

In order for you to start feeling better and losing weight, you must support your immune system. If you do this, your immune system and metabolism will function at a much higher level.

Immune system support means removing toxins from the body, eliminating food allergies/sensitivities, decreasing stress, and giving your body the necessary nutrients to support your thyroid and speed up metabolism.

Most people eat to the detriment of their health and slow their metabolism through poor food choices, which also downgrades the immune system.

Substances like alcohol, sugar, caffeine, refined grains, fruit juices, sodas, processed foods, fast foods, and nicotine all place excessive internal stress on all systems of the body, including the immune system.

Because you have hypothyroidism, there may be certain foods in your diet that make your immune system go haywire; and if they're removed from your diet, you'll feel more energetic and lose weight.

If you have hypothyroidism, your thyroid is not functioning at a high level—which means all major physiological systems controlled by the thyroid are not working right. It's as if everything slows down.

Think of your thyroid like a car battery; if it's removed, no other systems of the car will work. You can jump-start the car, which may get it running; but until the battery is charged or replaced, all other systems of the car that the battery supports will not run.

This is similar to your thyroid. All the systems that your thyroid supports are running at about half speed.

This includes your digestive system, hormonal system, detoxification system, elimination system, etc.

This is why you have such a wide range of symptoms, from dry skin, depression, cold hands and feet, to hair loss, constipation, mood swings, and low libido.

One of the solutions is to medicate with a synthetic form of thyroid hormone, which will result in better blood test results, but this treatment may not get rid of the symptoms you're dealing with because your immune system was not addressed.

Unfortunately, you can't replace your thyroid, but you can support your immune system so that it functions at a higher level.

One of the big problems with hypothyroidism is that a portion of thyroid hormone is produced by certain systems of the body and if they're not functioning correctly, it will complicate your condition.

Two examples are your liver and gastrointestinal tract. These two systems help convert a portion of thyroid hormone T4 to T3—and T3 is the active form of your thyroid hormone that the body uses.

So, if your thyroid isn't up to par, it may not be making enough T4. If only a small portion of T4 makes it to your liver and your liver is not functioning at a high level, it won't put out enough T3. If this form of thyroid hormone is low, it will result in symptoms.

A similar situation can occur with your GI tract. If there's an overgrowth of bad bacteria due to poor diet and antibiotics, it can stress your thyroid due to conditions like leaky gut syndrome.

Certain systems of your body depend on each other to produce hormones, chemical messengers, and enzymes that are reliant on thyroid hormone to function correctly.

It's very possible that your liver isn't working at a high level because it's overworked and sluggish from the burden of detoxifying all the harmful substances you put into your body, and from the chemicals your body neutralizes from the external environment.

A sluggish liver can cause a reduction in the active thyroid hormone.

Your liver is also responsible for breaking down the fat, protein, and carbohydrates you eat, and if it's sluggish—this can also cause slow metabolic processing.

If your liver and GI tract aren't functioning right, chances are they might not be able to produce the substances they need to produce to help build hormones.

Can you see how diet can play a crucial role in hypothyroidism?

What you eat and drink fuels your body's systems so they are in-tune and not over-stressed.

Your body's systems are already running slow because of hypothyroidism, and the burden you place on them through stress, diet, and allergies makes the burden that much larger.

The right foods will ease the stress on the body so all the systems work at a much higher level. They will help organs produce hormones and enzymes needed to help your thyroid and hormonal system function correctly.

There are certain foods and elements that, when consumed in high quantity, can interfere with certain nutrients that feed the thyroid.

Also, there may be a certain level of nutrients needed for the thyroid to function that you may not be giving it.

In every case of hypothyroidism, there are modifications that can be made in the diet to help patients like you lose weight and feel much better.

This book will lay out all the foods that you should be consuming to make sure your thyroid isn't missing the important nutrients it needs to work properly.

It will show you the foods you should avoid that may interfere with hormone or thyroid production.

There will also be examples of foods that jack up your metabolism so you can lose weight easier.

There will be information about how certain beverages can make your condition worse and others that will help with weight loss.

Information will be provided on the best time to eat, how often to eat, how to pair your foods, and great spices to use that will help your metabolism.

Also, you will learn how to determine if your body doesn't respond well to certain food(s), and how to know if the meal you ate was right in terms of the ratio of macronutrients (fat, protein, carbohydrates).

One common question about hypothyroidism is, "What supplements can I take to help me lose weight with hypothyroidism?"

This is not an easy question to answer because everyone is different, everyone's response to supplements is different, and the causes of hypothyroidism are different. So, each cause may have a different treatment plan.

This book is not about how to treat the different causes of hypothyroidism. It is a nutritional program to support the immune system and help the body lose weight.

However, there will be suggestions on a few supplements you can take that will help just about anyone with hypothyroidism.

Remember, the purpose of a supplement is to supplement or aid your diet. And if you have a poor diet or you're not following the food plan, your results will suffer.

So, focus on food first, then supplementation.

Changing your diet alone will make a huge difference to how much weight you lose, and how you feel.

Diet is important for anyone who wants to lose weight, but especially important for hypothyroidism—because your body is operating differently from those without this condition.

You will have to make certain sacrifices in your diet so you can feel better and lose weight, but these sacrifices will seem small once you realize the benefits from making these changes in your diet.

In fact, you will probably wish you made these changes much sooner.

One thing to remember is once you have been told that you have hypothyroidism, particularly Hashimoto's, you can never reverse this condition.

This doesn't mean you won't get better—or you'll always struggle to lose weight, but it does mean you should never go back to your old dietary habits.

You can still enjoy sweet treats, specialty drinks, and meals on special occasions. But it's the reoccurring act of eating improper foods that stresses your body.

So, don't dwell on the things you can't have, instead try to enjoy the new foods you'll be introducing into your diet.

You are about to start a new journey, a journey of discovering about foods, your body, and how they interact. You'll learn things that most people don't know about food and nutrition. This knowledge can be very beneficial.

This new knowledge you gain can ensure a long life abundant with energy, free of disease and excess body weight, if you choose to use it.

—————————— *Chapter 1* ——————————

Hypothyroidism and Digestion

One of the major complications with hypothyroidism is how it affects the digestive system. The metabolic slow-down causes a number of digestive problems in patients with this condition.

Symptoms of sluggish digestion include bloating, indigestion, constipation, malabsorption, and flatulence.

These symptoms exist for a number of reasons...

Research has shown that people with hypothyroidism have lower levels of serum gastrin and other enzymes that are produced by the pancreas. Gastrin is responsible for the production of hydrochloric acid, which aids in the digestion of food in the stomach.

The reduction in HCL means that food will sit in the stomach longer and leave the stomach only partially digested. If the food leaving the stomach is only partially digested, it will make digestion more difficult during the next phase of the digestive process.

Another problem that occurs with digestion is that the contractions of muscles that move food along through the GI tract have become sluggish. This will decrease the transit time of food through the entire system.

As a result, food remains in your system longer and can result in bacteria overgrowth, fermentation, and constipation, which can cause further health problems such as Candida and Dysbiosis.

Also, if food is not fully digested—it means the body will be unable to fully absorb the nutrients available in the foods you eat. This could lead to other symptoms of hypothyroidism such as depression.

As you can see, when you have problems with your digestive system not only can it cause symptoms directly related to digestion, but it can also lead to other health problems and symptoms indirectly related to hypothyroidism.

Don't Overcook Your Food

I bet you can remember your mom telling you to eat your veggies when you were a youngster—hopefully you've listened and you've been doing it for years. Now, it's even more important, because there is a lack of vitamins and minerals in the foods you eat, especially the veggies.

There is a downward trend of nutrient depletion from what sits on your dinner table. The amount of bioavailable vitamins and minerals has been shrinking from decade to decade and, as a result, you now must eat twice the amount of fruits and vegetables to make up for what's missing.

The RDA for fruits and vegetables was a recommended five servings a day. Now, the servings have risen to 9-13 because of low nutrients in your food.

You can get some nutrients from fortified juices, milk, and cereals, but it just isn't the same. Taking a multivitamin will help if you choose the right one, but it's not as good as the real thing.

I am going to show you how to extract more nutrients out of the foods you're already eating, how to make the food easier to digest, and how to lose a few pounds in the process.

There is a book written by a famous dentist—his name was Francis Pottenger. Dr. Pottenger documented the results of a little experiment he did with some cats, which has had a huge impact on how we eat, or at least it should have.

Francis decided he was going to study how food affected people. Well in this case, cats.

He started with groups of cats similar in size, age, and health. He fed all the cats a similar diet—the only difference was that one group got cooked food, and the other ate raw food.

At the end of the study, the groups of cats looked completely different. The study took place over a few years and the amazing thing was the group of cats that ate the raw food was lively and vivacious, while the other group was burdened with chronic disease.

The only difference was the mere cooking of the food.

Now, my point is not that you become a RAW foodie. My point is, if you eat the same foods you have been accustomed to, but start preparing them differently, you could make a big difference in how you feel and look.

For example, let's look at meat. Americans eat a lot of meat, and most people eat their meat well done.

If you're a steak lover, have you ever felt full and bloated after eating meat?

One of the problems with cooked meat is that it is very hard for your body to digest.

However, if you eat meat that is medium rare instead of well done, it will be much easier for your body to digest and you'll get more nutrients from it because it hasn't been denatured through the cooking process.

Meat contains vitamins, minerals, and other nutrients such as enzymes. Enzymes will help break the meat down naturally if not destroyed through cooking. The enzymes actually help digest your meal.

You will get more nutrients out of eating meat and your body will be happier if you don't cook it all the way through. You don't have to eat it raw, which may involve some risks, but just try eating it a little less cooked than what you're accustomed to.

Another misnomer is that you should eat all your veggies raw to get all the nutrients from them.

Well, not so fast.

Did you know that you have to cook carrots to 104 degrees Fahrenheit to extract the beta carotene from them? Otherwise, all you get from raw carrots is fiber.

The fact is the body doesn't contain a cellulose enzyme that is needed to break down the fibrous part of veggies and to extract all the nutrients. In order to get the most out of your veggies, you should cook them just a little bit.

I'm not suggesting that you overcook them until they're mushy. Just cook them enough until they are al dente—still a bit crunchy, but not hard.

Most people, because of their digestive system, find it very hard to digest raw veggies, and cooking them slightly will make a big difference.

If you have no problems with digesting food, feel free to eat some raw veggies. A good rule of thumb is to have a variety of both raw and cooked veggies at every meal.

How to Make Digestion Easier

Because your GI system is not like that of others—and it runs at a slower pace, you must change some things about how you eat if you want to lose weight and feel better.

It amazes me that very few doctors address the diet of patients with hypothyroidism, even though digestive difficulties are a symptom of the condition.

The good news is you can help your digestive system by taking stress off of it just by doing some simple things. You may not even have to drastically change your diet.

First, it may be helpful to know a little about how digestion works, so you can take the steps needed to make things easier for your body.

Digestion begins in your mouth, and just by making a concentrated effort to chew your food more before you swallow will make digestion easier.

Your mouth contains an enzyme called amylase. This enzyme helps digest carbohydrates. The more you chew, the more you stimulate your body to produce this enzyme and the more this enzyme mixes with the food.

This may sound a little silly, but try counting how many times you chew your food before you swallow. Then, try increasing this number to 25-30. This simple step may help reduce your symptoms.

Also, this little tip will help you to not overeat.

Another simple thing you can do to help digestion is to drink more water.

Because of the decreased transit time of food through the GI tract, more water is extracted from the food, making it hard and difficult for defecation.

More water will help with digestion by softening the stool.

Also, water helps produce certain fluids of the body that help with digestion. These are the same fluids that you may have a limited amount of because of hypothyroidism. These fluids include enzymes and hydrochloric acid.

The body relies upon water to produce these very important digestive aids—so drink more water in between meals.

Notice I did not mention to drink more water with your meals and there is a reason for this.

Your body works very hard to break down the meals you eat, and if you drink a lot of fluids with your meal, it will make the process more difficult. You may be thinking that drinking fluids with meals helps with digestion, but the opposite is true.

Drinking a lot during the meal actually dilutes the acid and enzymes needed to break food down. This makes the digestive process longer and harder on the body because the body will need to produce more digestive juices to get the job done.

It's ok to drink with your meal, but try sipping instead of gulping down fluids. Drink just enough to enjoy the taste of your drink or to rinse your mouth, but don't use it to wash your food down.

The best time to drink is in between meals when there is no food in your stomach.

Also, be sure not to drink too much just before the meal or right after your meal. Allow 20 minutes before and after your meal before slugging down beverages.

Food Combining

The way you eat can be very stressful on your digestive system and if you have hypothyroidism, your digestive system is already running at half speed.

Your food choices with every meal greatly impact how easily and how fast your meal will be digested.

Thanksgiving dinner is a great example.

Think about how you feel after Thanksgiving dinner...you probably feel bloated, gassy, and tired. Often, it's not because you ate too much, it's because you have eaten heavy starches and heavy proteins together. This is very difficult for your digestive system to break down.

The food will sit in your stomach for a long time until it is digested. Plus, because it's very hard on your digestive system, it requires a lot of energy—so you get tired.

Instead, try to eat your protein with your veggies, or eat your carbohydrates with your veggies, but don't mix a heavy carbohydrate and a heavy protein.

Other great examples include steak and potatoes, hamburger and French fries—you get the idea.

It has been suggested that when you eat protein like meat your body produces a certain acid to digest it, and when you eat a starch like potatoes your body will produce an opposing acid to break it down. And when these opposing acids mix, it makes it harder to break the food down.

As a result, the food will sit longer in your stomach and the body will produce more acid, trying to get the job done. This process is hard work for your digestive system.

So, if you want to feel light after your meal and avoid bloating, fullness, and gas, try eating protein with veggies and your starches with your veggies and try to avoid mixing your animal protein and starchy carbs.

One of the problems with having hypothyroidism is that your metabolic rate has fallen, which causes your digestive system to slow down. Eating this new way will help your digestive system break down food much faster and easier.

This will lead to less digestive upsets and constipation. And...your body will be getting more nutrients—and the more nutrients your body gets, the less hungry you'll be and the less food you'll crave. Also, this process will help you lose weight.

The Most Powerful Digestive Aid

What I am going to suggest to you next is so simple and powerful, that it allowed one patient to stop his prescription medication for indigestion.

Unfortunately, you now live in a world of go-go-go. You're probably unaware of the stress you're under from day to day because you don't pay attention to your body.

What you don't realize is that subtle and constant stress on your body causes a stress response inside of your body, and these reactions can have an impact on your digestion.

One of the worst times to eat is when you're under stress. When you're under stress, the body will direct blood flow away from the stomach to areas of the body that require it in a stressful situation, like your brain and extremities.

Just think of yourself being chased by a pack of wild dogs...you don't really need blood in your stomach at this time, do you? Wouldn't you rather have the blood, oxygen, and energy delivered to your legs and brain instead?

Your stomach is not an area of the body where you need blood in a stressful situation. Yet, you probably eat under stress all the time.

If you eat when you're on the go and under stress, the food in your stomach will sit there like a rock until the stress response has subsided.

Eating under stress can cause indigestion, bloating, and gas.

So, before you eat your meal, make sure that you sit down to eat—don't stand!

✡ Then, once you're sitting down, take ten deep breaths—inhale through your nose and exhale out through your mouth. Try to inhale and exhale as slow and deep as you can. Make the inhalation to a count of seven and the exhalation to a count of fourteen. When you exhale, purse your lips.

This simple exercise will force oxygen into the stomach along with blood supply by reducing the stress you're under—and helping you digest your meal faster and more efficiently.

Also, doing this simple breathing exercise before you eat every meal will make your meals more enjoyable to eat.

Eat Like Europeans and Lose Weight

One group of people that follow this technique indirectly is the Europeans. They take long lunches; they eat slowly—enjoy conversation, family, and friends and most often they'll walk to and from their lunch.

Another way to de-stress when you eat is to change your mindset. For instance, try to pretend you're on vacation...

I know you probably feel that's impossible to do—but try it, because there are many cases of people actually losing weight on vacation because there was no stress and they ate casually.

This will allow you to burn up your meals quickly and easily.

This lifestyle has contributed to a lower rate of chronic and preventable diseases all over Europe. Plus, it helps shrink the waistline.

Also, the simple act of adding some movement into your day, such as walking after meals, will also help digest your meal, not through burning calories—but by helping your digestive tract move food along through the intestines.

✡ Remember, your digestive motility rate has slowed, so movement around your midsection through walking, twisting, flexing or extending the torso will help move food along faster.

Add Veggies and Get Skinny

Another thing you can do that will help you lose weight and make digestion easier on your body is to add more veggies to your diet.

A good rule of thumb to follow is to never eat a meal without vegetables.

Veggies will help lower the calorie content of your entire meal; veggies will add fiber, vitamins, minerals, and water to your diet.

The fiber in vegetables will help draw water to the food being digested—and as you know, water is very important for digestion. And most veggies already contain a healthy portion of water.

Fiber also helps control blood sugar, as it will not allow your blood sugar to spike after a meal. And ultimately, controlling your blood sugar is a key factor when trying to lose weight.

Adding veggies to your meals is a win-win scenario. Pick out a group of veggies that you like and make sure to stock up on them so they are always available in your refrigerator.

Another easy way to get more veggies into your diet is to start planning your meals around vegetables, not meat—if you eat meat.

Vegetables are also great as snacks. Just make sure to pick vegetables that are not part of the goitrogen family and try to choose non-starchy vegetables for your meals and snacks.

Starchy vegetables are veggies that are high in sugar, like peas, corn, carrots, and potatoes. Also, the more you cook starchy vegetables, the more sugar they will contain.

There is a whole chapter dedicated to goitrogens later in the book.

Also, there is a full list of great vegetables in the meal planning section that will not harm your thyroid or blood sugar.

Digestive Supplements

One of the best digestive aids that you can use to help make digestion easier on your body is found in the produce section of your local supermarket. Not only is it easy to find, but it's also cheap.

I'm talking about lemon!

You're probably getting a sour taste in your mouth just thinking about lemon, but you don't have to eat it, so don't worry.

The acid in the lemon will help kick-start your body to produce stomach acid, which helps digest your meal.

Here's what you need to do...

About 20 minutes before your meal, squeeze a large lemon wedge into an eight-ounce glass of purified water, make sure the water is room temperature before you drink.

This will help kick-start the body's own digestive mechanism.

Another thing that you can do to help with digestion, if you're having trouble, is to take one of two digestive supplements.

The first one is called betaine hydrochloride.

This is very similar to the hydrochloric acid found in your stomach. Most people over the age of 50 have a lower output of acid compared to young adults.

First, use the lemon to see if it helps, then proceed by taking hydrochloric acid if you're still having digestive troubles.

The other supplement that can be easily found in health food stores is a digestive enzyme.

The main ingredient in this supplement is a proteolytic enzyme called *bromelain*. This is the same enzyme that is found in a certain part of pineapple. It will help digest the protein in your meal.

Protein is one of the hardest macronutrients to digest, and when you combine it with fat and a complex carbohydrate it can make digestion very difficult, especially if consumed in large quantities.

These are just a couple of helpful hints to help with your digestion and absorption. If you can't digest your food properly, you won't be able to use the nutrients found in the food.

Always remember, focus on food first, then supplementation.

Action list

- **Chew your food**
  Make an effort to chew your food more when you're eating. Count how many times you chew before you swallow. Increase the number to 20 – 30 repetitions.

- **Breathe**
  Make sure you're not under stress when you eat. Make a point of sitting down for meals and take 10 deep breaths before eating.

- **Water**
  Increase the amount of water you drink in between your meals. Don't drink 20 minutes before or after meals.

- **Movement**
  Include some form of movement after your meal to help with digestion.

- **Eat your veggies**
  Eat vegetables with every meal. Plan your meals around what veggies you're going to eat. Keep pre-cut veggies in your refrigerator for snacks.

- **Drink lemon water**
  Squeeze a large lemon wedge into eight ounces of purified room temperature water and drink 20 minutes prior to a meal.

- **Add a supplement**
  Try supplementing your diet with betaine hydrochloride or digestive enzymes to help digest your meal.

- **Food combining**

Combine either protein with your vegetables or complex carbohydrates with your vegetables. Do not eat heavy proteins with complex carbohydrates, e.g. steak and potatoes.

Resources

Books:

The SlowDown Diet: Eating for Pleasure, Energy, and Weight Loss, Marc David

Nourishing Wisdom: A Mind-Body Approach to Nutrition and Well-Being, Marc David

Supplements:

Betaine Plus HP, Biotics Research. www.bioticsresearch.com

Bromelain Plus, Biotics Research. www.bioticsresearch.com

Chapter 2

Halogens

This is not your high school chemistry class, nor do I want it to be, but do you remember the periodical table hanging on the wall in your science class that you had to memorize?

Well, now would be a great time to recall this chart. There was a section on the table for a group of elements called halogens.

The halogens are bromine, chlorine, fluorine, iodine, and astatine.

What do the halogens have to do with your thyroid?

Well as you now know, iodine is part of this group of halogens and it is also the major mineral and nutrient responsible for the health of your thyroid.

The problem is that the rest of these halides have no place in the human diet and are very damaging and toxic to human biochemistry, yet all humans have a heavy load of these halides inside their body.

The health of your thyroid becomes compromised when the rest of these halides compete with iodine and displace it from where it needs to go—your thyroid.

You see, some of the halogens are similar in shape, yet some are larger than iodine. And when it comes time for the body to absorb iodine, it may absorb the other halogens instead because of their size and iodine is being outnumbered.

The standard American diet (S.A.D.) is almost completely absent of iodine because of farming trends, soil depletion, the absence of table salt utilization, and the lack of iodine rich foods in the SAD.

Because of the low level of iodine in the SAD and the increase of other halogens entering the body, your body is thirsting for this mineral.

To help your thyroid, you can increase iodine absorption and utilization by eliminating or reducing the other halogens and increasing your iodine intake.

How to Get More Iodine

There are two ways to increase your iodine intake: diet and supplementation.

I recommend that you get your iodine from natural food sources not supplementation.

Supplements show inconsistent results because of unregulated supplements and the inability for patients to test iodine levels on their own.

Also, I DO NOT recommend that you use iodine supplements because supplementation with iodine has been documented to initiate Hashimoto's thyroiditis.

You can have a genetic marker for hypothyroidism, yet you might not have the condition because it hasn't been "turned on."

Iodine supplementation has been documented to stimulate hypothyroidism and all its nasty side effects.

Too much iodine can cause your immune system to go into attack mode on your thyroid.

So, supplementation with iodine can sometimes do more harm than good.

Instead, consider increasing your iodine intake through diet.

One easy way of increasing your daily intake of iodine is to use sea salt. However, buyers, beware!

It seems everyone today is selling sea salt because it's supposedly more natural and healthier than plain table salt. However, most of the salt produced has been modified and denatured—and some brands don't even contain iodine.

This is where label reading becomes important.

You may be asking why salt is processed, and the answer is so it can sit on the grocery store shelf longer, so it looks better, and it's easier to use.

Companies use aluminum as an anti-caking agent in salt so it doesn't stick together, and other companies use sodium chloride, which can cause issues with high blood pressure.

The bottom line is, you want fresh *Celtic* sea salt. This type of salt is still wet when you buy it, and you'll need a grinder to break it up for consumption. There's a recommended company in the resource section.

You can add some sea salt to your food, and if you drink water throughout the day, I recommend putting some in your water. 1/4 teaspoon in pure water twice a day is sufficient.

If you use good sea salt, you will not only benefit from the iodine in the salt, but it also contains over 80 other minerals that your body can use. This is better than most mineral supplements.

Iodine-Rich Foods

Other ways of getting iodine into your diet is through food rich in iodine. Most ocean fish are primary sources of this trace element. Fish are able to extract and concentrate iodine from sea water.

Here is a list of foods that are high in iodine.

- **Seafood**
  - Cod
  - Shrimp
  - Tuna
  - Haddock
  - White deep water fish
  - All varieties of shell fish
  - Fish oil
- **Sea weeds**
  - Kelp
  - Wakame
  - Nori

- **Vegetables**
  - Spinach
  - Turnip green
  - Swiss chard
  - Summer squash
  - Lima beans
  - Garlic
- **Milk products**
  - Yogurt
  - Condensed milk
  - Cheddar cheese
- **Eggs**
- **Mayonnaise**

How to Reduce Your Halogen Exposure

Now that you're up to speed on where you can get your daily dose of iodine, let's focus on how you can reduce your exposure to the rest of the halogens.

Other halogens that you may come in contact with daily are bromine, chlorine, and fluorine.

The first two, bromine and chlorine, go hand in hand when used to treat the water you drink, shower in, or swim in. They are used to disinfect and kill bacteria found in water sources.

You can't stop drinking water or showering, but what you can do is filter the water you use to drink and bathe in to reduce your exposure to chlorine.

Just to demonstrate that you're drinking chlorine if you're not filtering your water, try this little test...

Fill a glass of water and let it rest for a day to release some of the chlorine from it. Next, fill a glass from your tap. Smell both water glasses and taste.

Chlorine from tap water has been known to evaporate if it is left out and not refrigerated.

This is not a recommended way to reduce chlorine in your water. This is just to point out that this nasty halogen is in the water you drink.

There are numerous companies that make water filters. Do some research and find one that filters the halogens bromine and chlorine or check the resource section of this book.

Shower filters are also widely available. Also, there are companies you can send your water to for testing, Doctor's Data is such a company. Check the resource section for their contact information.

One thing to keep in mind is that your skin is the largest organ on your body and it contains a lot of blood vessels. So, anything you put on your skin gets absorbed into your blood stream. Some hormone replacements are in the form of a cream because it is better absorbed through the skin.

The point here is, when you shower in steaming hot water your blood vessels will dilate and easily absorb the chlorine in the water that is all over your body. Not to mention, these chemicals become more concentrated when heated through the steam.

So not only are you showering your body in chlorine and bromine, but you are also inhaling it. You could also be inhaling fumes from the products you clean your shower with, like bleach and ammonia.

Other sources of bromine include bromine-based fire retardants used in carpets, mattresses, upholstery, furniture, and electronic equipment. Bromine is a suspect for causing a number of medical conditions, including hypothyroidism.

Don't Swallow Your Toothpaste!

The other halogen widely used is fluorine, and the obvious place to look for fluorine is in your toothpaste. But it can also be found in your drinking water.

Fluoride should not be in anything that you're putting into your body. If you read the toothpaste label for toddlers, you'll notice that it doesn't contain fluoride, and your toothpaste with fluoride will suggest you don't swallow it.

In fact, most toothpaste tubes have warning labels on them.

Have you ever wondered why this is?

Most of Europe has outlawed the use of fluoride in their drinking water. This is because in large quantities it can do some major damage to your biochemistry.

Fluoride is also found in some medications. Prozac is loaded with fluoride and it can be found in many others. Make sure you inquire with your pharmacist if you're taking any prescription drug.

There is a great book on fluoride and I suggest you read it—the title can be found in the resource section.

Rocket Fuel in Mama's Milk?

Another man-made chemical to keep an eye out for is perchlorate. Perchlorate is another chemical that competes with iodine, and its widespread pollution is causing health problems and awareness.

It can be found in water, produce, and milk—but it's not supposed to be there.

Perchlorate is made and used for car airbags, leather tanning, fireworks, and rocket fuel. And unfortunately, it is ending up in the breast milk of new mothers.

If you're a mother and you're breast-feeding your new born, isn't it scary to think you could be feeding your infant rocket fuel?

There are stories like this making news in local communities all around the U.S.

Dangerous chemicals like perchlorate end up in the foods you eat and the beverages you drink every day.

The best defense against these chemicals is to increase your awareness.

The good news is your body has a detoxification system, but you do have to help your body in this battle. The bad news is not all these nasty chemicals actually make it out of your body.

A lot of chemical bi-products get stored in the fatty tissue of the body.

And it's the overload of toxic substances that disrupt the internal environment of the body that can cause hormone confusion, which may lead to conditions like hypothyroidism.

One detoxification method for removing halogens from the body is through adequate iodine intake.

When your body is supplied with enough iodine, it will rid your body of the other dangerous halogens that it doesn't need.

This is just another reason to make sure that you are getting enough natural iodine into your diet through food.

Start increasing your iodine consumption through food and drink to detoxify your body from these substances and protect your health and thyroid.

Checklist

- Increase iodine consumption through food.
- Reduce exposure to harmful halogens.
- Use only filtered water for drinking and showering.
- Use toothpaste and food products free of fluoride.

Resources

Books:

Iodine: Why You Need It, And Why You Can't Live Without It, Dr. David Brownstein

SALT Your Way To Health, Dr. David Brownstein

The Fluoride Deception, Christopher Bryson

The Case Against Fluoride, Paul Connett

Water Testing:

Doctor's Data Inc. www.doctorsdata.com

Water Filters:

Nikken www.nikken.com

Chapter 3
Goitrogens

There is some concern surrounding a certain group of foods called goitrogens, which may cause goiter or the enlargement of the thyroid. Goiter is caused through suppressing the thyroid function by interfering with iodine uptake.

However, there are some things to consider before you skip the produce section of your grocery store because this is where most goitrogens are found. As you can guess, goitrogenic foods are largely a group veggies, fruits, and nuts.

My guess is that your thyroid condition did not arise from an over consumption of these healthy, cancer-fighting foods.

It's true, if you consume a large quantity of raw goitrogenic foods, it could lead to problems.

However, if you're like most Americans, you probably don't live on a diet strictly composed of raw fruits, nuts, and seeds.

Plus, most goitrogens can be inactivated through cooking.

However, because you do have a thyroid problem you want to do everything you can to help out your thyroid, so it can function better and so you can feel better.

The goitrogens that you want to pay particular attention to are the ones that you often eat in a raw state. They may be fruit and nuts, or certain veggies.

If you eat raw goitrogens often, you should reduce your consumption. Also, try cooking them. If they're the fruit and nuts you like, make substitutions.

For example, if you like peanuts and peanut butter, try almonds and/or almond butter. If you like strawberries, try blueberries or raspberries. You get the idea.

Another way around this is to pay attention to what you eat and drink and try to vary and rotate your foods. Remember, too much of one food is never good for you. Eat everything in moderation and with balance.

Try not to eat the same foods more than 2-3 times per week.

Also, beware of goitrogens that you eat often—but you're unaware you're eating them because they're hidden in the ingredient labels of the packaged food you buy.

This is one more reason to start reading food labels.

The Truth About Soy

One particular goitrogen that is found in many, many foods that you should be on the watch for is soy.

Soy has been ordained as a noble health food and medicine. At the same time, it is downgraded as a food substance that promotes hormonal disruptions in the body and cancer.

There are entire books written about this subject and some of the information is worth reading, it may open your eyes to how soy affects your body.

Soy is everywhere and used for everything. Soy is in your make-up, it's in your food, and it's in the food that feeds livestock and fish. And the real problem with soy, other than the fact that you can't get away from it, is that it is highly processed.

Most of the soy you consume is probably in oil form, which is used to make breads, crackers, and other processed foods.

So, how do you get away from it?

You can't.

All you can do is limit its consumption by being aware of it. Soy

If you're a vegetarian and consume artificial meat products made with soy—try to cut it out. If you use soy sauce—cut it out. If you eat tofu—limit how much and how often you eat it.

Some researches say that the fermented forms of soy are ok to eat. However, because you have hypothyroidism you should limit your consumption.

Another area where soy is found in abundance is in nutrition and energy bars. Soy nuts are used as the main protein source in most meal replacement bars.

Just because something is labeled as *healthy* and it's a nutrition product doesn't necessarily mean it's good for your body.

Remember, there are very few companies that are in the business of keeping you healthy. The bottom line for most companies is profit margins—and profit margins are increased through cheaper ingredients.

The best way to reduce the consumption of soy is just by increasing your awareness. So, start reading labels of everything that you put in or on your body.

The Real Problem with Soy

One of the big problems with food today is mass production. When foods are mass produced, the natural process of growing food is altered—which leads to a not-so-natural product, and your body pays the price.

There is concern about how genetically modified (GM) foods may affect the human body, and 91 percent of soy grown in the U.S. is GM.

GM foods are created to resist certain toxic herbicides—so this means that the soy you eat is loaded with nasty chemicals. Also, soy is GM from a different gene that produces a protein that your body may not recognize. Because of this fact, there has been an increase in allergies to soy.

Once this gene enters the intestines of your body, it can harvest there and you can continue to have allergies to soy even after you stop eating it. Also, research has shown that this allergy can be passed down through generations.

Soy contains a substance called hemagglutinin, which causes your red blood cells to stick together, and when this happens you're unable to fully absorb oxygen and deliver it to the rest of your body.

Soy also contains "anti-nutrients" called phytates. Phytates prevent your body from absorbing certain minerals like calcium, magnesium, iron, and zinc—and as you may know, you need these minerals to help build bones, fight off infections, and for energy.

Along with phytates, other "anti-nutrients" in soy include saponins, soyatoxin, protease inhibitors, oxalates, and estrogens. Some of these interfere with the body's ability to digest protein.

As you can see, soy contains quite a few "anti-nutrients" along with other harmful substances. But one of the biggest culprits is estrogen.

Soy is loaded with isoflavones, which is a type of phytoestrogen, meaning it looks a lot like the real estrogen your body produces. When you consume these phytoestrogens, they can mimic the real estrogen or block the absorption of estrogen, which can lead to hormone disruption, infertility, and even cancer.

If you're a woman, drinking just two glasses of soymilk a day for one month provides enough of these compounds to alter your menstrual cycle.

Peanuts

Did you know that peanuts are actually a legume? And the problem with peanuts is that they contain lectins and other anti-nutrients that can adversely affect your health, particularly if you're suffering from an autoimmune disorder like Hashimoto's.

The anti-nutrients in peanuts can interfere with your body's absorption of vital minerals, some of which your thyroid needs to function.

Some say that these anti-nutrients can be neutralized through roasting, but the jury is still out—and if you have hypothyroidism, you should minimize your consumption just to be cautious.

This also includes peanut butter. Peanut butter not only contains roasted peanuts, but most major brands will add trans fats in the form of hydrogenated oil to make spread easier, and salt and sugar to make it taste better.

Another problem with peanuts is that they contain *aflatoxin*. Aflatoxin is a potent human carcinogen produced from mold that infests peanuts and other crops like corn, wheat, rice, and soybeans. Peanuts are among the top three crops that are affected by aflatoxin.

In order to control the growth of this mold, farmers will spray peanut crops heavily with herbicides—another reason to reduce consumption.

Lastly, peanuts have a tendency to cause allergic reactions to those who eat peanuts and/or peanut butter, especially to children.

A good substitute for peanuts and peanut butter is raw organic almonds and almond butter.

Dangerous Oils

Did you know that the cells in your body are composed primarily of saturated fat? This type of fat gives your cells a rigid, yet flexible cell wall to allow the good stuff in and the bad stuff out.

By the way, saturated fat is the type of fat everyone is warning you to stay away from so you don't get heart disease. It's found in animal fat, cheese, and butter.

However, what scientists are now finding out is that it's not the saturated fat that is causing the problems.

The fats that are the REAL problem are unsaturated fats, particularly polyunsaturated fats.

These fats include corn oil, soybean oil, safflower oil, and sunflower oil. These fats remain liquid at room temperature.

What makes these oils so bad is that they are very unstable and easily turn rancid. These are mainly store bought oils in clear plastic containers. Some manufacturers will add antioxidants in the form of other oils in hope of protecting the oils from going bad.

These oils are very sensitive to heat and light.

You should purchase oils in dark glass bottles that are cold pressed and organic. Store your oils in your refrigerator.

The fats you should use for cooking are coconut oil, butter, and olive oil.

Olive oil and butter are good to use while cooking over moderate to high temperatures, and coconut oil is best for high temperature cooking.

The reason why these fats are better for cooking is that they have a higher smoking point and are more stable.

Olive oil's best use is for salads, and it is referred to as monounsaturated fat. When you use olive oil for salads, you can enjoy the natural fruit and nutty flavors that come from the oil.

You can also stir-fry and light cook certain foods in water and then add olive oil to the cooked foods for taste.

Getting back to the danger of fats...the reason why polyunsaturated fats are so bad is because they affect the cell structure, and sometimes the body won't even recognize the cell.

This causes miscommunication in the body and disrupts hormonal balances, which leads to endocrine problems such as hypothyroidism.

Fat is also needed to make the hormones in your body, and if your body is not getting enough of the right kind of fat, it will also lead to hormone imbalances.

As you can see, the fat in your diet is extremely important and often overlooked.

Once again, start reading labels and try to avoid as many of these bad oils as you can.

If you're using canola or any other oil for cooking or dressings, make the switch to coconut and olive oil.

Other Goitrogens...

Other goitrogens to watch out for are any fruits, nuts, seeds, and vegetables that you eat often and eat raw.

These might include pears, strawberries, peaches, peanuts, and pine nuts.

If you like any of these, try to cut down your consumption or make substitutions for them.

If there are veggies that you eat often and they're part of this group—make sure you cook them.

Here are additional goitrogenic foods to watch out for.

Goitrogenic Foods

- Soybeans (and soybean products such as tofu, soybean oil, soy flour, soy lecithin)
- Pine nuts
- Peanuts
- Millet
- Strawberries
- Pears
- Peaches
- Spinach
- Bamboo shoots
- Sweet Potatoes
- Bok choy
- Broccoli
- Broccolini (Asparations)
- Brussels sprouts
- Cabbage
- Canola
- Cauliflower
- Chinese cabbage
- Choy sum
- Collard greens
- Horseradish

- *Kai-lan* (Chinese broccoli)
- Kale
- Kohlrabi
- Mizuna
- Mustard greens
- Radishes
- Rapeseed (*yu choy*)
- Rapini
- Rutabagas
- Turnips

Checklist

- Go through the list of goitrogens and put a check mark next to the fruits, nuts, and veggies that you eat often; this will help increase awareness.
- Either replace your favorite foods with alternatives or reduce your consumption.
- Make sure you're cooking the vegetables on this list and rotate your menu so that consumption of any one vegetable is no more than two to three times per week.
- Replace your peanut butter with organic almond butter.
- Check food labels on processed snacks, dinners, and nutrition bars for soy content. Find a replacement!
- Throw out all of your cooking and salad oils and replace with organic cold pressed extra virgin olive oil, coconut oil, and raw organic butter.

Resources

Books:

The Whole Soy Story: The Dark Side of America's Favorite Health Food, Kaayla T. Daniel

Know Your Fats: The Complete Primer for Understanding the Nutrition of Fats, Oils, and Cholesterol, Mary G. Enig

---

Chapter 4 ---

Hidden Sugars That Make You Fat

This chapter is focused on a substance/food that if removed from your diet would completely change how you feel and look.

In fact, if sugar was removed from the American diet, there would be very little work for doctors and pharmaceutical companies.

Sugar is what makes food taste good and it's probably what you crave. The only other cravings that may tempt you are salt and fat. And if you were to satisfy your craving with fat instead of sugar, you would be better off.

I know what you're thinking...if I eat fat, I will get fat and fat is not good for me.

Well, I have news for you; you need fat and without it you would become depressed, achy, fat, and miserable and you would eventually perish.

There are good fats and bad fats and if you replace the sugar you eat with good fats, your body will thank you.

Fat is responsible for many building blocks in the body such as hormones, cells, and nervous tissue.

However, this chapter is not about fat, but I will tell you that eating the wrong type of fat is the second biggest culprit to health problems, just behind eating too much sugar.

More on fat later...let's focus on the sweet stuff.

Sugar comes in many forms, and when you think of sugar you probably think of candy, cookies, cake, baked goods, soda, and the pure white granulated stuff that you put in your daily cup of joe.

However, these are just the obvious forms of sugar that you're already aware of.

Sugar is any substance that your body uses to increase your blood sugar quickly.

For instance, did you know that white and wheat bread turns to sugar in your body within thirty minutes after eating?

There is a whole category of food that has this same action on the body, but it's disguised to be healthy food on the shelf at your local super market.

One way of distinguishing foods that cause a rapid rise in blood sugar is to follow the Glycemic Index. This will help you avoid eating foods that are too high in sugar.

Other foods that break down quickly into sugar within the body include things like pasta, breads, white rice, crackers, and most processed foods.

The processing of food removes most of the nutrients so that it can have a long shelf life.

In some cases, food may be fortified with nutrients that were taken out. And these are also foods you want to avoid.

When in doubt about what you're eating, always remember—stay as close to nature as possible and ask yourself this...

Did man make it?

If so, it's best to avoid it.

This same philosophy was adopted by the late legendary fitness guru Jack LaLanne, who has recently passed at the age of 96.

Is Fruit Making You Fat?

Another popular form of sugar that you may be consuming and thinking that it's good for you is fruit and fruit juice.

This is a controversial statement, but I stand by it.

For the average person, a moderate consumption of fruit may not be harmful to their health. However, others who have health issues, such as diabetes or other conditions related to obesity, should avoid fruit and fruit juices like the plague.

Also, for anyone who is looking to lose weight and/or reduce body fat fruit and fruit juice should also be avoided.

One of the problems with fruit is that most fruit has been genetically modified to taste sweeter. Companies are doing this for obvious reasons, and there is more sugar in fruit today than there was decades ago.

Some fruit is better for you than others, and there will be a full list of the fruits to avoid and the fruit you can consume moderately later in this chapter.

It's true that there are some fruits loaded with certain vitamins, minerals, and the popular buzz word antioxidants.

Recently, there has been a rage about the tiny dark fruits from far-off rain forests that have been suggested to cure every problem under the sun.

I'm sure you have heard of gogi berries, wolfberries, and acai.

These fruits are not much better than the fruits available at your local market—so, save your money on the magic juices.

Some of the best fruits to consume are berries. These are the fruits that are loaded with antioxidants, and they're the same fruits that have been around for millions of years.

These include blackberries, blueberries, boysenberries, strawberries, raspberries, and cranberries.

Just make sure you eat these in moderation and try to buy organic.

These berries are mass produced and heavily sprayed with herbicides and pesticides. Herbicides/pesticides place a toxic load on the body, and if you have hypothyroidism, you want to avoid further toxicity.

In fact, research shows that toxicity of certain pesticides/herbicides, heavy metals, and other environmental pollutants have a large contributing factor to hypothyroidism.

There are entire books dedicated to these topics, and if you have hypothyroidism, it's wise to investigate how you can avoid contact with them.

Sugars to Avoid

Getting back to sugar...

Your body doesn't know the difference between the table sugar you put in your coffee and the sugar from an apple. The only difference is how fast it is absorbed—which is dependent on the amount of fiber in the fruit you're eating, and any additional nutrients the body can extract from the fruit and other foods eaten at the same time.

Some of the better fruits to eat are those that contain higher amounts of fiber, such as apples and grapefruit. Fiber slows the digestive process, so your blood sugar doesn't skyrocket.

Other forms of sugar that are thought to be good for you and that I suggest you avoid are sugar substitutes like saccharin, aspartame, and sucralose. These sugars do not have a direct impact on your blood sugar, but studies have shown they have adverse side effects on the body when consumed regularly.

Even the natural sugar substitutes, such as agave, honey, and molasses, have a negative impact on blood sugar, and if you're trying to lose weight and control your blood sugar, it would be best to avoid them.

And of course, one of the worst sugars to consume that is found in just about every processed food available is high fructose corn syrup or HFC.

It's amazing that you can find this substance in hot dogs, bread, jellies, and many foods that you may not think would contain fructose. Just turn over any product in the super market and read the ingredient label.

Fructose has been associated with numerous health conditions, and some authorities suggest it is the main culprit for diabetes. Be on the watch-out for fructose!

Are you catching onto the hidden sugars in food and how you really have to pay attention and read labels to avoid them?

Sugar in Vegetables?

Believe or not, there are hidden sugars even in your vegetables!

No, I am not going to suggest you avoid eating vegetables, because they're a big part of this program and they're something you should eat with every meal.

But there are certain vegetables that do have a high amount of sugar, especially after being cooked. They are referred to as starchy vegetables.

These include potatoes, sweet potatoes, carrots, peas, corn, and squash.

If you have children or you can remember back to when you were a child, the veggies most consumed by kids belong to this group.

Can you guess why?

Of course...they contain more sugar, and kids love sugar.

This is not to say they don't have nutritional value, it's just that if you want to lose weight, body fat, or have blood sugar problems, they should be limited in your diet or paired with fats and proteins.

There will be a list of some of the best veggies to eat on this diet, and the veggies you should avoid when trying to lose weight.

Stop Drinking Sugar!

One of America's favorite beverages and a drink that is consumed worldwide is one that also raises your blood sugar indirectly.

Can you guess what it is?

This not an obvious consumer good that you would think would raise your blood sugar, but when consumed it gives you a sense of alertness.

It's coffee.

This may surprise you, and it does surprise most people that drinking a cup of coffee can raise your blood sugar.

It does this indirectly by initiating a stress response in the body.

The organ mainly affected by stress is your adrenal glands, and these glands produce a lot of hormones—one of which is cortisol.

Cortisol has many jobs; one of them is to make sure there is enough blood sugar flowing through your blood stream so that you have the energy available in stressful situations, some even life threatening.

Blood sugar is stored in your body in three places: your brain, your liver, and your muscles. And when your body gets a signal from cortisol, it will release blood sugar.

So, when you're under stress and you combine that with lots of caffeine and foods that are processed, you will continually have blood sugar instability, which can lead to adrenal, thyroid, and weight problems.

There are entire books written about caffeine and some of its negative side effects.

You'll find some suggested reading on this topic in the resource section.

Just remember, too much caffeine will raise your blood sugar, and too much blood sugar leads to health problems and weight issues.

Other drinks that contain lots of sugar include sports drinks, soda, diet soda, commercial smoothies, fruit juices, flavored coffees and teas, and alcohol.

Even milk contains sugar, but most of the sugar has not been artificially added to the milk if it's organic whole milk.

Hopefully, a light bulb is going on in your head, and you now realize how you may have been sabotaging yourself all this time by consuming hidden sugars in your diet.

The best way to avoid sugars in your diet is to become a label reader.

Sugar and Hypothyroidism

So, why is sugar so bad for you, what impact does sugar have on the body, and why does sugar impede the weight loss process?

You already know how it affects your adrenal glands, and there is a direct correlation between stressed-out adrenal glands and thyroid problems.

In fact, two major causes of hypothyroidism include blood sugar irregularities: insulin resistance and hypoglycemia.

Insulin resistance is when your body loses the ability to push glucose into the cells of the body with the help of insulin because the body is desensitized to insulin from the chronic exposure to glucose.

In other words, your body is ignoring insulin because it always wants attention—and this is a result of you eating too much sugar all the time.

Symptoms include fatigue after meals, constant hunger, craving for sweets—especially after meals, frequent urination, increased appetite or thirst, difficulty losing weight, aches and pains.

Hypoglycemia is low blood sugar. This occurs when you eat something high in sugar and the body produces too much insulin, causing your blood sugar to fall rapidly. When this happens regularly due to diet, the body cannot keep your blood sugar stable.

This will lead to hormonal disruptions, stress on the adrenal glands, the pituitary, and the thyroid.

Symptoms include craving for sweets, irritability from missing meals, caffeine dependence, light headedness from missing meals, eating to gain energy, shaky/jittery feeling, agitation and nervousness, becoming upset easily, poor memory/forgetfulness, blurred vision.

If you compare the symptoms of hypothyroidism with those of insulin resistance/hypoglycemia—don't they look somewhat similar?

This is one reason to reduce stress, caffeine, and sugar in your life.

Your body is affected by sugar in a number of different ways, most of which are negative, at least when sugar is eaten in excess and by itself.

All the negative reactions occur and snowball once the body has adequate reserves of sugar stored as fat.

Here's How Sugar Makes You Fat...

Let's say you eat something sweet, like a donut with a cup of coffee. Within minutes, the body starts to break down this simple form of sugar—which results in raising glucose (blood sugar).

When your blood sugar is elevated, your body needs to do something with this sugar, so your pancreas releases insulin to help the body move the sugar out of the blood and into the cells of your body.

And now that you have sugar in your cells, you have quick-energy and you feel pretty good, if not a little peppy from your sugar high.

The problem is, eventually your blood sugar will fall because your body has pulled the sugar out of your blood and put it elsewhere.

When your blood sugar starts to plummet, things start to happen...

You start feeling hungry again, you start to crave food—most likely sugar, you start to doze off and get sleepy. Your body's natural action is to keep you up/alert, and the way to do that is to reach for something sweet to bring your blood glucose level back up.

Now think if you consumed sweets with every meal, and your blood sugar and body was reacting this way all day long.

Well, this is how millions of Americans live and eat.

The problems really get bad once your body is no longer sensitive to insulin and you need more and more sugar to feel better. This eventually leads to diabetes and other lifestyle conditions like heart disease.

But before diabetes hits, the body goes through stages of storing sugar if your body is not burning it through exercise.

The body saves all this sugar for a rainy day, and it stores sugar as fat all over the body; your midsection (belly fat), around your organs (visceral fat), and in your arteries (triglycerides).

So, as you can see, sugar causes problems and a whole host of problems, other than being a little overweight and carrying that spare tire around your midsection.

The best way to avoid all this is to avoid sugar and all of the hidden sugars you now know about.

You're probably beginning to think this diet is not for me, it's too tough, and I can't live this way.

Not true!

How to Dampen the Sugar Effect

I am going to show how you can avoid cravings, mood swings, shrink your midsection, and skyrocket your energy levels.

It's ok to cheat once in a while and have a slice of pie, or some cookies, but the problem is *how frequently you do this, and how you combine your foods, and your choice of foods.*

The last sentence is the key to blood sugar stabilization, weight loss, and avoiding energy swings. It's more important than how many calories you consume or how big your portions are.

Here's why...

You can actually have some carbs in your diet, but the key is to limit the portion, and always eat carbs with other foods, especially fat and protein.

If you do this, your blood sugar will not react adversely, and the reaction won't be as severe as eating something like a candy bar all by itself.

Try to forget about calories for a moment, just focus on how your body works in regards to your blood sugar.

The more sugar you put into the body at once and by itself, the quicker and higher your glucose level will rise.

But if you combine sugar or carbs with fat and protein in a meal, your blood sugar won't spike because of the fat and protein.

So remember this...

The most important thing to do when eating something sweet—if you have to, is to combine it with fat and protein. This way, it won't cause a spike in your blood sugar.

<u>Also, start to think of everything you eat as a meal...even your drinks.</u>

Have you ever noticed how quickly a person can get intoxicated when drinking alcohol on an empty stomach?

Well, this happens because the body has nothing else to process, and the alcohol goes right from the blood stream and into your cells.

But if you eat something while drinking, it takes longer to process and the immediate reaction isn't as bad.

So never, ever, eat something sweet by itself when you're trying to control your blood sugar and your weight.

Another little trick to help melt off the fat is to add up all the carbs in a meal and compare it to the fat and protein in the meal.

Think Pie!

Do not eat a meal when the portion size of carbs is larger than the fat portion or the protein portion.

Think of your meal like a pie chart with equal portions of carbs, fat, and protein.

Your body is completely different from everyone else's, and you require different ratios of protein, fat, and carbs, but use this pie chart as a general rule of thumb.

The nice thing is you don't have to weigh food, count calories, or points.

<u>But remember, you have to consider the beverages you drink and the desert in the meal as the total amount of carbs for that meal.</u>

So, include your juice, alcohol, bread, deserts and/or pasta from a meal to your carb portion and compare that to your fat and protein in the meal.

If you're overloaded or heavy on the carb portion, cut out some carbs until it's balanced.

And when you're trying to lose weight, your carb portion should be smaller than the portion of fat — or protein.

If you visualize this, you can see how easy it is to go overboard on the carbs and get into trouble with your weight.

Here's a helpful tidbit when it comes to actual portion sizes.

As a general rule of thumb, try not to have any portion of macronutrients— that is, the size of the carbohydrate, fat, or protein portion on your plate exceed something you can hold in one hand.

Keeping your portions smaller will ultimately help you lose weight, and it also makes it easier on your body to digest your meal. And if you have hypothyroidism, your metabolic rate as well as the rate at which your body processes food will be slower than most.

Anything you can do to take stress off the body will help your condition.

Do Your Homework

Ok, here's your homework...

I mentioned in the beginning of this book to approach it as a plan and program just like a prescription from a doctor. The value in this book is by DOING, not just reading.

If you follow this, you'll be successful and see results much quicker. Plus, you'll be able to follow this plan as a lifestyle, not just a quick weight loss diet.

Here's what you need to do...

Write down everything you eat and drink during the day for an entire week. This is not hard to do and the best way to do this is to carry seven 3X5 note cards with you and a pen.

After you finish a meal or drinking something, write down in detail what you ate or drank and document the time you did it.

Do this every day for a week because your eating habits will probably change on the weekend.

At the end of each day, sit down with this book and your note card. Use the reference section at the end of this chapter and identify the carbohydrates you ate for the day. Then, compare those numbers to the numbers of better choices you could have made and will make in the future.

This is one of the best ways to learn.

However, don't read the charts and meal plans yet. Eat as you normally eat and then come back to the chart and see where you could have made better choices.

Also, you need to look at each meal or drink and compare the portion size of carbs to the portion size of fat, and protein.

The key here is to be able to identify all the carbs, even the hidden ones and compare the portion size to the other macronutrients like a pie chart.

If you're like most people, you have the habit of eating the same things, which is not good. But it will allow you to identify some of the sneaky carbs in your diet and catch on quickly to how many carbs you're eating with every meal.

Once you start reducing your carbs and pairing your carbs with protein and fat, you will begin to notice a difference in your energy and the weight will slowly start to melt off.

Glycemic Index

High GI Foods   =   GI of 70+ (Try to avoid. Keep as a reward.)

Medium GI   =   GI of 55 to 69. - (Use with caution. Avoid when possible.)

Low GI   =   GI of 0 to 54. - (This is your target zone. Choose foods with a low GI value.)

Category	Food Name	Glycemic Index
Vegetables	Baked Beans, 4oz.	48
	Kidney beans, 3 oz.	27
	Lima beans, 3 oz.	32
	Navy beans, 3 oz.	38
	Pinto beans, 4oz.	45
	Soy beans, 3 oz.	18
	Beets, 3 oz.	64
	Tomato Sauce	49
	Peas	48
	Sweetcorn	48
	Broccoli, cauliflower, celery	10-25
	Vegetarian chili	39
	Mashed potato, instant	74
	French Fries, baked	54
	Potato, peeled & steamed	65
	Carrots	47
Breads	Dark rye, 1.7 oz.	51
	French baguette, 1 oz.	95
	Hamburger bun, 1 bun	61
	Kaiser roll, 1	73
	Pita bread—whole wheat, 1 slice	57
	Sourdough, 1 slice	52
	Fruit Bread	53
	White bread, 1 slice	70
	Wonder Bread, White Enriched	71
	Wheat bread—stoneground, 1 slice	53
	Whole wheat, 1 slice	69
	Bagel, plain, white, 2 oz.	72
	Wholegrain Bread	40
	Multigrain Breads	45

	English Muffin, Whole Grain	45
	Oat Bread	65
	Rye Bread	50
	Bran Muffin	65
Meats / Chicken	Sweet & Sour Chicken w/Noodles	41
	Lean Cuisine, French style Chicken	36
	Beef casserole	53
	Chicken Nuggets, frozen	46
	Fish Fingers (strips)	38
	Pizza, cheese	60
	Sausages	28
	Hamburger (with bun)	66
	Chicken Nuggets, frozen & microwaved	46
	Sushi, roasted	55
Cereal	All-Bran Kellogs, 1/2 cup	42
	Bran Flakes, Post, 2/3 cup	74
	Cheerios, 1 cup	74
	Cocoa Krispies, 1 cup	77
	Corn Chex, 1 cup	83
	Corn Flakes, 1 cup	84
	Corn Pops, 1 cup	80
	Cream of Wheat, 1 oz.	74
	Frosted Flakes, 3/4 cup	55
	Froot Loops	69
	Grapenuts Flakes, 3/4 cup	80
	Frosted Mini Wheats, 1 cup	58
	Honey Smacks	71
	Multi Bran Chex, 1 cup	58
	Muesli, 2/3 cup	43
	Raisin Bran, 3/4 cup	73
	Rice Chex, 1 1/4 cup	89

	Shredded Wheat, 1/2 cup	83
	Honey Smacks, 3/4 cup	56
	Special K, 1 cup	54
	Total, 3/4 cup	76
	Pancakes, from shake Mix	67
	Pop Tarts	70
Rice	Barley, pearled, 1/2 cup	25
	Couscous, 1/2 cup	65
	Instant, 1 cup, cooked	87
	Uncle Ben's, converted, 1 cup	44
	Long grain, white, 1 cup	41
	Short grain, white, 1 cup	72
	Rice Noodles	53
	Instant rice—white (boiled)	87
	Brown rice (boiled)	72
	Brown rice (steamed)	50
Cookies	Graham crackers	74
	Oatmeal cookie, 1 cookie	55
	Vanilla wafers, 7 cookies	77
Crackers	Rice cakes, plain, 3 cakes	82
	Stoned wheat thins, 3 crackers	67
	Water cracker, 3 crackers	78
Dairy	Ice cream, vanilla, 10% fat	61
	Low Fat Ice Cream	35
	Milk, whole, 1 cup	27
	Milk, skim, 1 cup	32
	Milk, chocolate, 1 cup, 1%	34
	Pudding, 1/2 cup	43
	Milk, soy, 1 cup	31

	Tofu frozen dessert, low fat, 1/2 cup	115
	Yogurt, nonfat, fruit, sugar, 8 oz.	33
	Yogurt, nonfat, plain, artificial sweet	14
	Yogurt, nonfat, fruit, artificial sweet	14
	Custard, 3/4 cup	43
Fruits	Apple, 1 medium, 5 oz.	38
	Apple juice, unsweetened, 1 cup	40
	Apricots, 3 medium, 3 oz.	57
	Banana bread, 3 oz.	47
	Banana, 5 oz.	55
	Cherries, 10 large, 3 oz.	22
	Cranberry juice, 8 oz.	52
	Grapefruit, raw, 1/2 medium	25
	Grapes, green, 1 cup	46
	Kiwi, 1 medium	52
	Mango, 1 small	55
	Orange, 1 medium	44
	Orange juice, 1 cup	46
	Peach, 1 medium	30
	Pear, 1 medium	38
	Pineapple, 2 slices	66
	Plums, 1 medium	69
	Prunes, 6	29
	Raisins, 1/4 cup	64
	Watermelon, 1 cup	72
	Cantaloupe	65
Pasta / Pizza	Fettuccine, 6 oz.	45
	Linguine, 6 oz.	52
	Linguine with Shrimp Dinner	40
	Macaroni, 5 oz.	47
	Deluxe macaroni & Cheese Dinner	36

	Ravioli, meat, 4 large	39
	Ravioli, durum wheat flour, meat	39
	Spaghetti, white, 6 oz.	41
	Spaghetti, wheat, 6 oz.	37
	Spaghetti, white, boiled	42
	Spiral, durum, 1 cup	43
	Tortellini, cheese, 8 oz.	50
	Vermicelli, 6 oz.	35
	Pizza, Super Supreme	36
	Pizza, Vegetarian Supreme (Pizza Hut)	49
	Lasagna, vegetarian	20
	Lasagna, meat (Healthy Living brand)	28
	Lasagna, beef	47
Snacks	Vanilla wafers, 7 cookies	77
	Doughnut, deep-fried	75
	Apple Muffin	48
	Sponge cake, plain, 1 slice	46
	Snickers, 2.2 oz. Candy bar	41
	Pretzels, 1 oz.	83
	Potato chips, 14 pieces	54
	French Fries, 4.3 oz.	75
	Popcorn, light, microwave	55
	Popcorn, regular	72
	Pop Tarts, chocolate, 1 tart	70
	M&M's Chocolate candy, peanut	33
	Snickers Bar	41
	Mars Bar	68
	Peanuts	14
	Cashew nuts	25
	Granola Bar, chewy, 1 oz.	61
	Graham crackers, 4 squares	74
	Doritos Corn chips, 1 oz.	72

Drinks	Coca-Cola, 1 can, 12 oz.	77
	Gatorade, 8 oz.	78
	Fanta soft drink, 1 can, 12 oz.	63
	Apple Juice	40
	Orange Juice	50
	Tomato Juice	38
	Lemonade, sweetened	54
	Fruit Punch	67
	Chocolate Milk	34

Checklist

- Start identifying the hidden sugars in your diet by logging a food diary for one week and reading foods labels.
- Follow the simple rule of never eating anything sweet or any carbohydrate by itself for a meal, snack, or drink.
- Compare the ratio of macronutrients; fat, protein, carbohydrate for every meal/snack. Visualize a pie chart.
- Make sure the portion of carbs for each meal is smaller than the portion of fat or protein when trying to lose weight.
- Compare the carbohydrate choices you made to better choices you could have made by using the glycemic index.
- Start thinking about what you drink as a meal and if you drink something sweet or something that contains caffeine—or alcohol, eat some fat or protein along with it.
- Keep your portion size of each macronutrient (fat, protein, carbohydrate) to the size of something that can fit in the palm of your hand.

Resources

Books:

Suicide by Sugar: A Startling Look at Our #1 National Addiction, Nancy Appleton

Lick the Sugar Habit, Nancy Appleton

Sugar Blues, William Dufty

Sugar Busters, H. Leighton Steward

Chapter 5
Food Allergies/Sensitivities

Sugar can be damaging to your health and it can jeopardize weight loss, but there is another food that can be just as bad as for you and worse than sugar if you have hypothyroidism.

You already know that processed grains are a form of sugar and they rapidly turn into sugar in your body.

It's this up and down seesaw effect of blood sugar that causes most of the health/weight problems.

However, processed grains not only cause disruptions in blood sugar— they also can be seen by your body as a foreign invader.

This foreign invader is what's known as an antigen and can cause severe problems to your immune system, which may result in damage to just about any part of your body.

When a food substance is seen as a foreign invader within the body, it causes an immune reaction referred to as a food allergy.

The difference between a food allergy and a food sensitivity/intolerance is that a food allergy usually causes an immediate and severe reaction that sets off your immune system to release a cascade of chemical messengers such as histamine.

Food sensitivities can cause similar reactions, but are usually milder and don't necessarily involve an immune system reaction.

Believe it or not, very few people have food allergies—less than eight percent of children under three, and less than four percent of adults.

Most reactions are intolerances not allergies.

Food allergies can cause immune reactions as mild as a cough to an extreme as a malfunction of the respiratory system, or have a delayed reaction or no noticeable reaction at all.

One of the problems with food intolerances is that you may not even know you have a problem even as you continue to eat the food, and most of the foods that cause sensitivities are ones you probably crave.

So you may be wondering...if I don't have a reaction to a food when I am eating it, yet I have sensitivity to it, can it really be doing me any harm?

The answer is yes.

It's not until you actually remove this substance from your diet for a period of time and then reintroduce the food that you may notice a reaction.

This is referred to as an elimination or provocation diet, and it's the best method for determining if you have a food allergy or sensitivity.

The most common food allergies include **eggs, soy, milk, peanuts, gluten, corn, and seafood.**

If you read the ingredient label on food packaging, you'll notice these common allergens are found in most prepackaged foods, with the exception of seafood. And if they're not in the food, they will most likely be processed on or with equipment shared by the rest of the highly reactive foods.

Avoid This One Food to Lose Weight and Beat Fatigue

One food allergen that has recently been shown to have a common connection with those who have hypothyroidism is **gluten.**

Gluten is the protein found in wheat, but the protein that actually does the damage is called *gliadin*. However, everyone else knows it as gluten, so it will be referred to as gluten in this text.

The connection between gluten and hypothyroidism is due to the molecular structure of gluten and thyroid tissue.

Scientists have discovered that the thyroid cell tissue and the gluten molecule are very close in structure. In fact, your body can't tell the difference between them.

If you have hypothyroidism, it's very likely that your body is inadvertently destroying your thyroid.

It's a common cause of mistaken identity, and here's how it happens...

When you become sensitive or allergic to any food, it's the protein found in the food you like and eat often that causes the problem.

During digestion, part of your food goes undigested and sneaks into your blood stream where it doesn't belong, and it's here where the identification of an antigen begins and so does the attack on the foreign invader.

Once this protein has been labeled as an invader, the body never forgets it. And it's important to know that if you have gluten allergy or intolerance, you should never eat it not even in small amounts.

It only takes one gluten protein molecule to set off an alarm in your body that there is an invader, and it can take up to six months to calm down the immune response that the allergen caused.

But how does this protein get into your blood stream?

It all begins with a condition called leaky gut syndrome.

Leaky gut (LG) is due to poor intestinal health—specifically the thinning of the epithelial tissue in the GI tract. This thinning has a number of different causes. It could be because of stress, too much sugar in the diet—which causes the cells in the tissue to separate and let the invader through, or it can come from overuse of over-the-counter pain medications or antibiotics.

Whatever the cause, it's important to recognize there's a problem and fix it before it gets worse.

It's not uncommon for people to have more than one food allergy at a time and in some cases, many.

It has been estimated that up to 81 percent of Americans have a genetic predisposition to gluten intolerance, with 35—50 percent experiencing some form of reaction. However, 8 percent of people don't even know they have it.

Gluten intolerance is becoming more and more common among both adults and children due to awareness, diet, processed food, and slow genetic modulation.

It's possible that once you fix the leaky gut problem your immune reaction may become absent. But eating gluten itself weakens the intestinal tract and leads to the destruction of your thyroid. So, the risk of eating gluten may not be worth it.

Everyone has different reactions to food sensitivities and the symptoms can range from a cough and congestion, itchy red skin flare-ups, stomach upsets, headaches, bloating and gas, to muscle aches, joint pain, confusion, mood swings, and dizziness.

The thing to remember is that you have hypothyroidism and that your reaction is different from others who don't have hypothyroidism, because your body can actually be destroying thyroid tissue every time you consume gluten.

What Foods Contain Gluten?

Unfortunately, this is not such an easy question to answer because there are lots of obvious foods that contain gluten—and there are some very "unassuming" food products and condiments that contain gluten as well.

One reason there is an increased number of people affected by this food allergy is the processing of food.

Gluten is used in many products and condiments as a binder, filler, to add texture, for thickening, as a flavor enhancer, and stabilizer.

Gluten is everywhere and hard to avoid. And when you realize just how common gluten is—it's easy to understand why it causes so many problems.

The best way to start identifying gluten is to start reading the ingredient label on **ALL** food products you want to buy. This may seem a daunting task at first, but with time you will know what contains gluten and what doesn't without reading a label.

Do you see a common trend between trying to find the hidden sugars mentioned earlier in this book and trying to identify gluten?

The bottom line is, you have to start reading labels and understanding what you're putting into your body.

Our food has changed over the past few decades—and there continues to be more added ingredients into the food system because of technology advancement.

In fact, most of the vegetables and fruits you consume are genetically modified, they're referred to as "frankin foods" you know, just like Frankenstein.

A good rule of thumb to follow is, if the food you're going to eat wasn't around one thousand years ago—don't eat it!

And even though grains were available back then, it wasn't until 10,000 years ago that grains were brought into the food chain.

One of the arguments about grains is that we were not genetically made to eat grains and that our genetics haven't quite caught up to the way we currently eat. This can be another reason for celiac disease and gluten intolerances.

How to Find Gluten in Your Food

The easiest way to start identifying gluten is to think in terms of flour—and what products are made with flour.

The basic grains you need to avoid are wheat, barley, and rye. However, there are hybrids of wheat that you also need to avoid which include spelt and kamut. Also, remember it's anything that is made with or from these grains, such as malt which is derived from barley.

Start identifying the basic gluten products with this list...

Gluten-Containing Foods

- Bagels
- Biscuits
- Bread
- Bread crumbs
- Breaded fish
- Breaded meats or poultry
- Bread pudding
- Cake
- Cereal
- Chicken nuggets
- Croissants
- Cookies
- Crackers
- Croutons
- Doughnuts
- Dumplings
- Flour
- Flour tortillas
- Fried vegetables
- Ice cream cones
- Macaroni
- Melba toast
- Muffins
- Noodles
- Pancakes
- Pasta
- Pastries
- Pie crusts
- Pizza crust
- Pretzels
- Rolls
- Spaghetti
- Stuffing
- Tabbouleh

- Waffles
- Graham crackers
- Hamburger buns
- Hotdog buns

These are just examples of major food items that you may encounter.

Foods You Wouldn't Expect to Have Gluten

You probably weren't surprised to learn that cakes, cookies, and all the other floury snacks contain gluten. After all, they're made primarily of wheat flour. The following list, on the other hand, may surprise you. These are foods that *usually* or *often* contain gluten.

In some cases, wheat is added as a thickener; barley malt is often added as a form of natural flavor. You must read the labels of these items carefully to look for gluten-containing ingredients. Even better, look for products specifically labeled gluten-free.

- Beer
- Beverage mixes
- Bologna
- Candy (many candies are gluten-free, so read labels)
- Canned baked beans
- Cold cuts
- Packaged cereals, even corn cereals
- Commercially prepared broth
- Commercially prepared chocolate milk
- Commercially prepared soup
- Custard
- Pudding
- Root beer
- Syrups
- Salad dressing
- Soy sauce
- Vegetables with commercially prepared sauces
- Custard
- Fruit fillings

- Gravy
- Gum
- Hot dogs
- Ice cream
- Non-dairy creamer
- Potato chips

Ingredients with Hidden Gluten

The tricky part is recognizing hidden gluten. By law, wheat must be clearly identified on labels. If wheat is listed, you know you can't eat the food. Unfortunately, wheat-free doesn't equate to gluten-free, and the law doesn't currently require all forms of gluten to be listed. Since barley, rye, oats, and their derivatives are all natural foods, they can sometimes be listed under fairly innocuous sounding names. That's why everyone with celiac disease or gluten intolerance, including children, must learn to recognize sources of hidden gluten. Study the ingredient list of all prepared foods and avoid those containing:

- Barley
- Binders
- Blue Cheese
- Bouillon
- Bran
- Brewer's yeast
- Bulgur
- Cereal binding
- Chilton
- Couscous
- Durhum
- Edible starch
- Emulsifiers
- Farina
- "Fillers"
- Hydrolyzed plant protein
- Hydrolyzed vegetable protein
- Kamut
- Kasha

- Malt
- Malt flavoring
- Malt vinegar
- Matzo
- Modified food starch
- Monosodium glutamate (MSG)
- Natural flavor
- Rye
- Seitan
- Textured Vegetable Protein (TVP)
- Wheat
- Wheat protein
- Spelt
- Soy sauce
- Stabilizer
- Suet
- Teriyaki sauce
- Semolina
- Some spice mixtures

There are foods like oats that do NOT contain gluten. However, during processing oats may be cross-contaminated with gluten, so it is usually on the do-not-eat list.

With time and practice, you will understand your body's reaction to gluten. Some people have major reactions and in others it may be mild. Also, you may not have a noticeable reaction to gluten, but the best way to identify this reaction is by removing it from your diet and then reintroducing the food after two weeks.

There will be more information on how to do this in the chapter on detoxification.

Gluten Alternatives

The good news is, because of the awareness of gluten allergies, substitutes for gluten are more and more common and can be found in most grocery stores.

No longer is there need for specialty shops solely for providing gluten-free products. Costs have come down and the taste from gluten-free foods has gotten much better.

However, if you don't care for the foods you're finding in your local grocery store, you can purchase baked goods from gluten-free bakeries and online.

Gluten intolerances have gotten so common that most foods that don't contain gluten are labeled on the front of the package.

But before you start grabbing packages and trusting food companies with your health, you should be aware of the alternatives for gluten.

Also, if you do a lot of your own cooking—which I strongly suggest, you should understand what you can use as a gluten substitute.

Here is a list of gluten alternatives...

Safe Replacement Flours and Starches

Grains flours / starches	Legume flours	Seed flours	Tuber flours / starches	Nut flours
Rice Corn Sorghum	Soy Chickpeas Fava bean Peanut	Flaxseed Millet Buckwheat Amaranth Quinoa	Potato Tapioca Arrowroot Sweet potato	Chestnut Almond Walnut Filbert

Even though the name buckwheat suggests that it may contain wheat—it is a safe alternative and does not contain gluten.

Getting Started...

Now that you know what you can eat and what not to eat, the key is to follow through.

Getting started is always the hardest part...

To help you on this journey, I have listed a number of websites and books available as resources and guides.

Once you recognize the effects of gluten on your body, how you feel, and the benefits from removing it from your diet, you'll be very reluctant to ever eat it again.

Remember, the most important thing is to try to replace gluten with all natural foods and not other processed foods that use gluten alternatives.

Most processed foods are loaded with man-made fillers and are very high on the glycemic index. These foods will cause blood sugar irregularities.

It's ok to eat these foods once in a while, but ninety percent of the time you should stay away from them.

Checklist

- Use your food diary from the previous chapter's homework and go through all the foods and mark the foods that contain gluten. Again, this will help create awareness.
- Next, look through the lists in this chapter for alternatives for the foods you marked in your food diary as containing gluten.
- Try to replace gluten-containing foods with **natural,** <u>unprocessed</u> foods.
- Go through your refrigerator and kitchen cabinets and identify any foods that MIGHT contain gluten and replace those with non-gluten products.

Resources

Books:

Living Gluten-Free For Dummies, Danna Korn

The Gluten Effect: How "Innocent" Wheat Is Ruining Your Health, Drs. Vikki & Richard Petersen, D.C., C.C.N.

Websites:

www.celiac.com

www.GlutenFreeWorks.com

Chapter 6

Jumpstart Your Metabolism

Water

One of the most important foods to consume is water. Now, you may not consider water a food, but water does allow your body to make use of the food you eat—and the food that is stored inside your body.

Let me tell you how important drinking water is for both weight loss and hypothyroidism...

Water is in every cell of your body, and in the compartments of what's called intracellular fluid, extracellular fluid, and plasma. It's the major component of blood and muscle. It helps the body detoxify itself; it keeps your body cool in the summer, and it's how different systems of the body communicate.

Water is important for so many reasons, and it also helps you lose weight.

Did you know that the brain triggers your thirst response and hunger response at the same time? So, you may think you're hungry at times, but it may actually be the thirst mechanism kicking in.

Did you know that your body is less hungry when you metabolize or break down fat and you can only metabolize fat with water? And you can't break down fat if you're dehydrated. This also means you will not be able to use fat as energy. So, being dehydrated can cause low energy levels.

You may also have low energy levels when under stress. This is because the brain constantly requires blood sugar—or energy, and the demand is higher under stress. The body has readily available stores of sugar, but it must be transported and transformed through water. And when the body is dehydrated, it will ask for more energy by triggering your hunger/thirst response.

It's not hard to see why people under stress eat a lot, so instead of eating under stress drink water.

Drinking water will increase your energy and reduce fatigue—and fatigue is a major symptom of hypothyroidism. Want more energy? Drink more water.

Drinking more water also helps you lose weight by substituting beverages like soda or juice for pure water.

There are documented cases of weight loss of 35, 40, and even 58 pounds in a year just from making the switch from juices and soda to water.

Not only are soft drinks these empty calories, but most of these drinks are loaded with sugar. And as you know, sugar causes many problems if you want to lose weight by disrupting your normal insulin cycle.

The only other beverages that you should be drinking regularly other than water are herbal teas, green tea, and vegetable juices. If you opt for vegetable juices, try juicing the vegetables yourself to reduce the sodium from commercial juices.

Here's how to tell if you are drinking plenty of water. When you urinate, the color of your urine should be a light yellow to clear. If your urine is dark yellow to orange, you need to drink more water.

Start by drinking a full glass of pure filtered water upon waking in the morning. This ensures that you get a good head start.

Why drink water first thing in the morning?

Because during sleep you slowly dehydrate yourself.

There's a little experiment I would like you to try—you've probably done this before as a kid. Put your face up against a piece of glass or mirror. Then, exhale out through your mouth to steam up the mirror.

What you're actually doing is exhaling water out of your lungs. And guess what...you do this all night long as you sleep—and throughout the day.

So, the best time to catch up on your water intake is first thing in the morning.

There are some authorities that may suggest you drink 64 ounces a day of water, others give you a formula based on your weight. The important thing is to increase your awareness as to how much you're drinking, and make more of an effort to drink more water.

Drinking more water will help you lose weight, beat fatigue, reduce headaches, reduce hunger pangs, decrease aches/pains, and help your immune system.

Fat

If you're like most people, you probably avoid fat like the plague, especially if you're trying to lose weight.

Unfortunately, fat has gotten a bad reputation over the years as a food that will make you fat, clog your arteries, and give you high cholesterol and a heart attack.

Fortunately, this is not necessarily true.

True, not all fat is good for you. In fact, a lot of it is bad for you, but what you may not know is that FAT is one substance that you need in order to lose weight and stay healthy.

Fat is what makes up every one of the cells in your body, it is the major substance of what your brain is made out of, it produces hormones, and the nervous system. Without it your body would break down and not function.

However, there is a big difference between good fat and bad fat, just like there is a big difference between good carbs and bad carbs.

The fact is, fat is a great source of energy and this is why your body stores energy as fat.

It should be a major component of all your meals because it will help you lose weight, create more energy, and balance your endocrine system.

However, you have to know your fats...

What you're going to learn is what type of fat you should and should not be eating, where to look for the bad fats and how to get more of the good fat into your diet.

Also, there is one type of fat that is known to help boost your metabolism by stimulating your thyroid.

Good Fats vs. Bad Fats

The obvious bad fat is the stuff that French fries, chicken wings, and egg rolls are cooked in. Some restaurants will use lard, but most restaurants buy cheap and highly processed oil that is no good for you which is soybean oil and or corn oil.

Anytime oil or other types of fat are heated to high temperatures to cook your food, or if your food contains a lot of fat and you cook it under high heat, it becomes very dangerous and harmful to your body.

Remember, fat makes up every cell in your body, and when you're putting bad fats in your body it makes your cells very rigid and hard. Cells should be flexible and allow nutrients and toxins in and out. Bad fats cause hormone disruptions in the body and it's one of the causes of hypothyroidism.

Another form of fat that is not good for you is the fat used in the processing of baked goods such as crackers or cookies. However, because of the awareness of trans fats, they are being removed from some store-bought foods.

Some of these fats are referred to as full or partially hydrogenated fat or oil.

This type of fat is found in foods like hot dogs, breads, cookies, crackers, peanut butter, and most foods that are processed.

Overall, it is very hard to find good man-made foods that are free of bad fats. This is why it is very important to avoid as many man-made products as possible.

When reading the ingredient label on packages, which you should start doing if you're serious about losing weight and keeping hypothyroidism under control, look for good fats such as olive oil, palm oil, and coconut oil.

Unfortunately, products containing these fats are hard to find.

The only processed foods you should eat are the foods you make in your kitchen because you can control the ingredients.

A lot of bad fats have entered the food cycle through farming. Most of today's livestock are being fed foods that are unnatural to them. Most animals eat a diet of corn and soy, which helps to fatten up the animals for selling.

For example, most cattle today are fed a diet heavy in soy and corn instead of grass. Grass is a natural source of food for cattle and when they eat off the land the cattle will produce a healthy form of fat known as omega 3.

I'm sure you've heard and are familiar with some of the health benefits of a diet rich in omega 3 fats.

A diet rich in sources of omega 3 fats can help fight depression, obesity, heart disease, and many other inflammatory diseases, not to mention these fats will help you lose weight.

Most animals today produce an omega 6 fat. The food you eat today is unfortunately loaded with omega 6 fats and not the healthy omega 3 fats. This is why fish oil supplements are a popular natural health food supplement— they are an omega 3 (good) fat.

One of the reasons why some fats are so bad for you is that they disrupt a normal hormonal balance within the body. And this balance is one of the reasons for hypothyroidism.

Bad fats cause inflammation, hormonal imbalances, immune problems, allergies, depression, and on and on and on.

Bad fats and sugar are the two most destructive substances that you can feed your body.

If you reduce or cut out unnecessary sugar and bad processed oils in your diet, you will start looking and feeling better.

The oils known as polyunsaturated fat acids are listed below and should be avoided both in food consumption and as a cooking medium.

- Corn
- Soybean
- Sunflower
- Safflower
- Cottonseed
- Canola

Because these oils are ubiquitous, they end up outnumbering the good oils in our diet and attach themselves to cells of the body, causing a disruption in communication and eventually disease.

One step towards losing weight is by balancing your hormones. This can be accomplished by removing harmful oils and sugar from your diet and replacing them with healthier options.

Start reading foods labels and avoid foods that contain the harmful oils listed on this page.

Remove these fats from your diet and replace them with good oils when cooking and making your own salad dressings.

Most oils are very unstable under high heat and most go rancid before they even make it to your kitchen this is another reason why they are bad for you.

Only buy cooking oil that is bottled in dark glass bottles. Make sure it's organic and minimally processed.

Extra virgin olive oil is a good oil to cook with under medium heat and it is very good to use in your salad dressings. Salad dressing is very easy to make.

Most commercial dressings are made with the other harmful oils mentioned and they should be avoided.

Another good fat to cook with under medium heat is butter. Opt for organic and preferably raw.

Kick-start Your Thyroid

Like most diets and nutrition information, coconut oil has been misunderstood and sometimes touted as a food that you should stay away from.

The main reason coconut oil has had a bad reputation is because it is mainly a saturated fat and some authorities and organizations have suggested that saturated fats will cause heart disease.

However, the history of coconut oil and its effects on the human body have never been documented to cause health problems.

In fact, it's just the opposite.

Coconut is loaded with vitamins, minerals, fiber, water, and fat. It is a great food, supplement, and cooking medium.

Coconuts have been used for thousands of years in many cultures for food and its health-healing properties.

Here is an excerpt from an interview done with one of the leading authorities on hormones.

In the 1940s, farmers attempted to use cheap coconut oil for fattening their animals, but they found that it made them lean, active and hungry. For a few years, an antithyroid drug was found to make the livestock get fat while eating less food, but then it was found to be a strong carcinogen, and it also probably produced hypothyroidism in the people who ate the meat. By the late 1940s, it was found that the same antithyroid effect, causing animals to get fat without eating much food, could be achieved by using soy beans and corn as feed.

Later, an animal experiment fed diets that were low or high in total fat, and in different groups the fat was provided by pure coconut oil, or a pure unsaturated oil, or by various mixtures of the two oils. At the end of their lives, the animals' obesity increased directly in proportion to the ratio of unsaturated oil to coconut oil in their diet, and was not related to the total amount of fat they had consumed. That is, animals which ate just a little pure unsaturated oil were fat, and animals which ate a lot of coconut oil were lean.

In the 1930s, animals on a diet lacking the unsaturated fatty acids were found to be "hypermetabolic." Eating a "normal" diet, these animals were malnourished, and their skin condition was said to be caused by a "deficiency of essential fatty acids." But other researchers who were studying vitamin B6 recognized the condition as a deficiency of that vitamin. They were able to cause the condition by feeding a fat-free diet, and to cure the condition by feeding a single B vitamin. The hypermetabolic animals simply needed a better diet than the "normal," fat-fed, cancer-prone animals did.

G. W. Crile and his wife found that the metabolic rate of people in Yucatan, where coconut is a staple food, averaged 25% higher than that of people in the United States. In a hot climate, the adaptive tendency is to have a lower metabolic rate, so it is clear that some factor is more than offsetting this expected effect of high environmental temperatures. The people there are lean, and recently it has been observed that the women there have none of the symptoms we commonly associate with the menopause.

By 1950, then, it was established that unsaturated fats suppress the metabolic rate, apparently creating hypothyroidism. Over the next few decades, the exact mechanisms of that metabolic damage were studied. Unsaturated fats damage the mitochondria, partly by suppressing the respiratory enzyme, and partly by causing generalized oxidative damage. The more unsaturated the oils are, the more specifically they suppress tissue response to thyroid hormone, and transport of the hormone on the thyroid transport protein.

Plants evolved a variety of toxins designed to protect themselves from "predators," such as grazing animals. Seeds contain a variety of toxins, that seem to be specific for mammalian enzymes, and the seed oils themselves function to block proteolytic digestive enzymes in the stomach. The thyroid hormone is formed in the gland by the action of a proteolytic enzyme, and the unsaturated oils also inhibit that enzyme. Similar proteolytic enzymes involved in clot removal and phagocytosis appear to be similarly inhibited by these oils.

Just as metabolism is "activated" by consumption of coconut oil, which prevents the inhibiting effect of unsaturated oils, other inhibited processes, such as clot removal and phagocytosis, will probably tend to be restored by continuing use of coconut oil. —**Ray Peat**

For more information on Ray Peat and his publications and/or services, go to www.RayPeat.com

As you can see, there are some great benefits from using coconut oil, especially if you have problems with losing weight and hypothyroidism.

Coconut oil helps the body by increasing metabolism, energy, and reducing the side effects of other bad fats that you may be consuming.

Remember, your cells are made up mostly of saturated fat—the same fat you get from coconuts.

If you can reduce the amount of bad polyunsaturated fats in your diet and increase the amount of saturated fat from coconut oil and raw organic grass fed dairy products and extra virgin olive oil, it will help your body's endocrine system function at a much higher level.

Start using coconut oil to sauté vegetables, use it in smoothies, use it in place of vegetable oil, and use it as a supplement for hypothyroidism and weight loss.

You can also use coconut meat and milk for various recipes. In fact, you can even use coconut flour as a substitute for regular flour in baked goods.

Start by adding two tablespoons of coconut oil to your diet daily.

Foods That Raise Your Metabolism

We've already mentioned two important foods that increase your metabolism, water and coconut oil, but there are many others that can stabilize blood sugar, raise metabolism and help burn calories all by themselves.

It is to your advantage to eat foods that can raise your metabolism, considering it's already running slow. Most of the foods, as you will see, are found in nature and are good for you.

One of these exceptions is caffeine.

Caffeine is a double-edged sword for those with hypothyroidism...

It can raise your metabolic rate, but it can also stress your adrenal glands, which can be a cause of hypothyroidism.

However, you can add caffeine to your diet in moderation from certain beverages once you determine that your adrenals are not overstressed and you have controlled your blood sugar.

Green Tea

When opting for caffeine, choose green tea. Green tea has less caffeine than coffee, and even less than decaf coffee. Plus, it's loaded with polyphenols—a form of antioxidant.

Green tea can also help with weight loss—but remember, everything in moderation. One to two cups a day should cause no harm.

Green tea can help increase your metabolic rate and add antioxidants to your diet.

A study in Switzerland discovered when the participants drank 2-3 cups of green tea daily it helped them burn an additional 80 calories. Make sure you don't add any sweeteners to your tea; otherwise you'll defeat its purpose. The tea helps the body burn calories through a process called thermogenesis. This means that the body will produce more heat; and when heat is produced, energy is expended and calories are burned. Also, green tea helps oxidize or burn fat.

The element in green tea that is responsible for weight loss is called epigallacatechin gallate or EGCG. This is the antioxidant in the tea that gives its green color. EGCG is also responsible for a host of other great health benefits like cancer prevention, cholesterol and blood pressure reduction, reduction of body fat and blood sugar, and protection against radiation, bacteria, and viruses.

If you don't like tea, there is good news. You can get green tea as a supplement. In fact, most weight loss supplements contain green tea or EGCG.

If you do opt for pills instead of the tea, look for a standardized extract of 60% EGCG. Doses should be in the range of 125-500 mg daily. This is the equivalent of 4-10 cups of green tea.

The best way to introduce green tea into your diet and to ensure better weight loss results is to replace your coffee, if you're a coffee drinker, with green tea. If you do this, you will be lowering your blood sugar and increasing the calories you burn at the same time.

Chili Peppers

Another food that can help you lose weight is chili peppers.

Have you ever eaten food so hot that it made your forehead sweat and nose run? If you like spicy foods, chili peppers are an excellent way of increasing your metabolism. They help you lose weight the same way green tea does—through the process of thermogenesis.

Isn't it great knowing that you can just turn up your body's furnace and burn more calories just by adding some spicy foods?

There is a family of chili peppers and they range from mild to super-hot. So don't think just because you don't like hot foods that you can't take advantage of this little fat burner.

You can add them to salsas, salads, fill them with cheese, roast them, and even make salad dressings from them. It's even easier if you buy the spice already dried and ground up so you can sprinkle it on your pasta, pizza, or chili.

Cinnamon

Cinnamon is an herb that has been used for thousands of years and has many health benefits, but was only recently discovered to aid in weight loss. It is the world's oldest known herb and has been used by the Chinese to treat numerous ailments such as nausea, diarrhea, and cramps. They have also used it to improve energy, vitality, and circulation. However, if you're looking for an advantage against weight loss, here is what we know.

Cinnamon's biochemical action that helps with weight loss is its ability to stabilize blood sugar. If your blood sugar is constantly rising and falling, you can bet that you will struggle with your weight. When your blood sugar fluctuates, you will have a tendency to crave sweet foods and your body will store excess sugar as fat. So, if you stabilize your blood sugar, you will start to feel better and look better, especially if you're exercising.

A recent study identified some health benefits of using cinnamon other than weight loss. The study's participants where those with type II diabetes who were asked to ingest ¼ teaspoon to 1 teaspoon of cinnamon daily for 40 days. After forty days, a measure of fasting blood sugar was taken and the participants lowered their blood sugar ranging from 18-29%. Also, their triglycerides fell 23-30%, LDL cholesterol fell 7-27%, and total cholesterol dropped 12-26%.

If you want to use cinnamon to help with weight loss, there are some important things to consider. First, not all cinnamon is made the same way. There are two common forms of cinnamon available. One is a baker's cinnamon referred to as Cassia, and the other is the real deal and referred to as Ceylon. Ceylon cinnamon is more expensive and harder to find, but worth the cost if you're focused on weight loss. Also, more is not necessarily better. There are certain elements found in cinnamon that can cause harm to the body when ingested in large quantities.

Cinnamon is a wonderful herb with lots of health benefits. However, to gain full advantage of it, you should use it consistently. Sprinkle it on your oatmeal, in coffee, or add to a casserole, but be sure not to overdo it. Remember, cinnamon is just one small advantage to the many you have against weight loss.

Other spices that help boost your metabolism include **anise, basil, cardamom, cumin, cayenne pepper, turmeric, garlic, ginger, chive, clove, coriander, fennel, nutmeg, and rosemary.**

Grapefruit

You've heard of the grapefruit diet and maybe you have even gone on the grapefruit diet. Well, eating grapefruit to help you lose weight is not just folklore, because it actually helps the body when trying to lose weight.

It has been suggested that this fruit contains fat-burning enzymes that will help you lose weight magically overnight, but it just doesn't work that way.

The fruit can help you lose weight because it is very low in sugar and contains a lot of fiber. Also, being low in calories, this fruit may help you lose weight by keeping your hunger under control through added fiber and water without the insulin spike. Plus, this fruit contains a lot of healthy vitamins and minerals.

There are other fruits that have a similar impact on weight loss, which include other **Citrus Fruits, Apples, Pears, and Bananas.** These fruits are low in calories and high in fiber. However, they have a bigger impact on blood sugar.

When you buy your fruit, make sure that it is organic, local, and fresh. You want to eat them just as they ripen, not after they have been sitting for days. Keep them in your refrigerator to keep them fresh. The longer a fruit ages, the more sugar content it produces.

It may be wise to eat only half of a piece of fruit if you really struggle with your weight. Choose bananas that are green tipped to eat, not the bananas with any brown spots because they will have more sugar.

Always eat your fruit with another source of complimentary protein, like nuts or cheese. This will keep your blood sugar from spiking.

For a variety, try adding some berries, which are loaded with antioxidants and polyphenols that fight disease. DO NOT USE DRIED FRUITS. Dried berries are LOADED with sugar and can delay your weight loss results. Keep your servings to a half of a cup.

Asparagus

Asparagus is a great weight loss food because it contains plenty of fiber, lots of vitamins such as vitamin C and folic acid, and it also has a diuretic effect on the body. So, it will help speed up the removal of metabolic waste and water through urination.

Because it is high in fiber and low in calories, it creates a zero caloric deficit—meaning it doesn't cost your body any calories to eat this food, because it takes more calories for the body to burn it up than the amount of calories in the food itself.

Other foods that have these same effects include **broccoli, cucumber, zucchini, spinach, greens beans, and garlic.**

Most green vegetables will have this action on the body, including veggies in the cruciferous family. Just be careful to cook them and limit your servings through each week.

Chicken and Beef

Lean proteins such as chicken and beef are great foods to include in a weight loss plan because of their thermal effect on the body.

Proteins are made up of branched amino acids that must be broken down into chains of peptides and reconfigured for usage in the body. The process of preparing proteins for the body to use is extremely inefficient, but good for weight loss because it requires a lot of energy. And of course, this energy translates into calories burned.

So, make sure to include three ounces of protein with each meal.

When eating meat it is always a good idea to eat all parts of the animal. There is protein in other parts of the animal, like the connective tissue. This may not sound appetizing, but you will get more nutrients from eating the whole animal instead of just the muscle.

In certain cultures, it's very common to respect the animal you're eating by using all parts of it. These cultures have proved that you will have better health if you eat everything.

Also, try to vary the meat sources you consume. Most meats contain a lot of tryptophan—which is an amino acid, and when it's consumed in large quantities it can suppress your thyroid.

Salmon

Another source of good protein and fat for your diet is fish. However, the fish I'm referring to is not so lean.

This is a fattier type of fish, but contains a good source of fat—Omega 3 fatty acids. As discussed earlier, this type of fat is needed in your diet. So why not get it through a natural resource like salmon. Other fish that also includes this good fat are **herring, mackerel, sardines, caviar, anchovy, and scallops.**

Shellfish

It is a good idea to rotate and vary your seafood sources as well. Other good fat and protein sources from the sea include lobster, shrimp, clams, crab, and muscles.

Avocado and Almonds

Although avocado is a fruit, it does contain mostly fat, the same as almonds, and both of these foods make great snacks.

Snacking on fat is a better option than snacking on most foods, because it has little impact on your blood sugar, it gives the body energy—because as you already know fat is a great source of energy; it's why the body stores fat.

Plus, it will satisfy your sugar cravings.

Other great snacks include hummus, hardboiled eggs, and dairy.

Hummus contains fiber and is great for dipping veggies.

Eggs are not thought of as a snack food, but they contain a complete array of amino acids needed for the body along with vitamins, minerals, and fat.

If there was such a perfect food, it would be the egg. You can have it at any time of the day, make it the main meal, and because it contains fat, it will keep you full.

Low fat dairy products are also good for a weight loss program, assuming you have no dairy allergies and/or sensitivities.

Milk and cheese contain a variety of amino acids and fat needed for the body. If you have a dairy allergy, you can use goat cheese and/or milk and buffalo cheeses. These products do not contain casein—the protein in milk that causes most allergy problems.

Other Ways to Stimulate Your Thyroid

Food is a great stimulator for your thyroid and metabolism when you choose the right foods. But it is also important when to eat.

Always eat breakfast to start your metabolism first thing in the morning.

Try to eat more frequently than you're used to. If you eat every five to six hours, make sure you snack in between meals—or try to eat your meals at four-hour intervals.

Also, another important element to help your body regain its metabolism is **sunlight.** Sunlight, as you know, is a great source of Vitamin D—which is actually a hormone needed for many functions in the body.

This is especially important during winter months. If you can't get out into the sun when it's cold, consider purchasing a light box that emits the similar light frequencies as the sun. This can help lift your mood, energy, and thyroid function.

One of the safest alternatives is to use full spectrum lighting in your house. This has many benefits without the risk of harmful rays.

Another source for raising your metabolism is exercise. This is a very sensitive activity for those with hypothyroidism, so I have included a chapter on this subject.

Please read and practice exercising according to the suggestions in this chapter.

Salt is important for those with hypothyroidism because it can help raise body temperature, improve sleep, help cells respond to thyroid hormone, and increase intestinal motility.

Use Celtic sea salt. Place a pinch of salt in drinking water first thing in the morning and just before retiring.

Checklist

- Increase your water consumption.
- Reduce your intake of polyunsaturated oils—corn, soybean, sunflower, and safflower.
- Increase your intake of saturated fat with coconut oil.
- Replace coffee with green tea.
- Eat breakfast and regularly throughout the day.
- Start using Celtic sea salt.
- Exercise regularly—especially resistance training.
- Make sure you get some sun in the winter.

Resources

Products:

Coconut oil — www.trpoicsbest.com

Sea salt — www.celticsealt.com

Books:

Caffeine Blues, Stephen Cherniske, M.S.

Salt You Way to Health, David Brownstein M.D.

Websites:

www.raypeat.com

Chapter 7

Do Supplements Really Work?

I wish I could tell you that all your prayers will be answered and your hypothyroidism will disappear, and you will lose 10 pounds overnight if you just take one little pill.

You have probably already been told something like this about a supplement you have bought or one that you've seen advertised on an infomercial, but the chances of getting results this dramatic just don't happen.

Supplements are great—and I am a big proponent of them, but they're not magic!

There's not one pill you're going to take that's going to change your body overnight or cure any problem that you have.

It's rare that you'll have a health problem that is a result of a single mineral or vitamin deficiency. These problems do exist, but this is not what you're dealing with.

Your problem probably exists because your body's systems are over burdened with too many stressors: chemical, physical, mental/emotional—and it can't handle all of them at the same time.

Generally, you can get great results by removing one food group from your diet and adding a supplement or two. But if you take the same supplement and you don't change your diet—your results will suffer.

A supplement is just that—it's a supplement to your diet.

So don't think that there is something out there that's going to change your life by popping a pill. A pill can never make up for poor lifestyle habits.

This holds true for most conditions and diseases.

Also, the research behind supplementation varies. You may hear from one resource that a particular vitamin is good for you and that it helps a certain condition, and another resource will tout the same vitamin.

This variation exists because all supplements are different—and of course, because of some special interest by the parties reporting the research.

Earlier in this book, I made mention that not all supplements are created the same way and therefore, the results will be different. Also, everyone's biochemistry is different so the result will also vary.

The key to getting good results with supplements is to make the necessary dietary changes, taking the right supplement in the right amount, and get a well-produced product with the right potency and without harmful byproducts.

If you don't know much about your condition—or about supplements, you'll have a hard time getting good results with supplements.

I am going to help you find the right supplements for you.

That being said, there will be some supplements that may help hypothyroidism, but will only work for a particular cause of hypothyroidism. So, the supplements that will be listed are those that can help everyone with hypothyroidism and weight problems without doing harm.

Please remember that more is not necessarily better.

For example, did you know that if you take large amounts of vitamin C for a long time, it can cause a copper deficiency? Or if you take large doses of zinc continuously, it can also result in a copper deficiency.

This can happen with all vitamins, minerals, herbs, and pharmaceutical prescriptions and non-prescription drugs.

It has been reported that all drugs have a minimum of 9 side effects and up to 500!

Think about that for a minute...

If you had good results from taking a drug, you wouldn't take more because it was working, would you?

The same holds true for any natural supplement.

Unless you have a good working knowledge on how to determine if you have a deficiency in a certain vitamin/mineral, or how to tell when you have taken too much of something, I suggest that you be more conservative with supplements versus being aggressive.

This book has been written to give you a blueprint of what to eat so you can lose weight with hypothyroidism. It is not designed to push pills or take short cuts. However, I've mentioned these supplements because they have been documented to help those with hypothyroidism.

Again, you will get better results from a change in diet and a couple of supplements, than not changing your diet and taking a lot of one supplement.

Supplements

The first supplement that I will mention is one that has been suggested to cure hypothyroidism, yet it can actually cause hypothyroidism symptoms when taken in excess!

Less is more in this case.

What I am referring to is iodine.

Iodine

If you look on the internet and search for a supplement that can help hypothyroidism, you'll find that most contain iodine. In fact, some only contain iodine.

Worldwide, the most common cause of hypothyroidism is a lack of iodine. The problem is, if you live in the U.S., you're not like the rest of the world...

Some parts of the world may be less industrialized and less advanced and may not have readily available sources of iodine.

Here in the U.S., iodine is easily accessible.

It's in the water, it's in the soil, it's in vitamin/minerals, it's in the salt, and added to formula for infants.

I am not saying that you can't be iodine deficient; what I am telling you is that in the U.S. the major cause for hypothyroidism is not iodine deficiency, it's Hashimoto's thyroiditis, which is an auto immune disorder.

So, if you have Hashimoto's or a genetic predisposition to hypothyroidism, yet you don't have any symptoms of the condition, you can turn on the symptoms with too much iodine!

The only way to know if you have a deficiency in iodine is to take a 24-hour urine sample test for the mineral.

Not all doctors run this test, and it is expensive.

The best solution, if you're not sure whether you're deficient or not, is to make sure you're getting iodine in your diet through natural sources like sea vegetables, sea food, and sea salt.

This way, it's very hard to get an excess of the mineral and cause an adverse reaction.

If you don't like sea foods, opt for sea salt and add it liberally to your foods and even to your water.

If you do decide to supplement with iodine use a combination of iodine and iodide, use the recommendation dosage by the manufacturer and make sure you test yourself.

Lugols is a reputable brand.

Tyrosine

Another nutrient that has been suggested to help hypothyroidism is the amino acid tyrosine.

Tyrosine is an amino acid that is necessary for the production of thyroid hormone. However, if your thyroid problem exists because of poor adrenal health—you can make your condition worse by supplementing with tyrosine.

In this case, tyrosine will reduce thyroid activity by over stimulating your adrenal glands which may already be over stimulated.

If you have a dopamine deficiency and you don't have adrenal insufficiency, tyrosine may help.

You can also make sure you are sufficient in the amino acid by testing.

Foods sources for tyrosine include chicken, turkey, fish, milk, cheese, yogurt, cottage cheese, lima beans, pumpkin seeds, avocado, almonds, and sesame seeds.

Selenium

Selenium is used in the body to help create more of the active thyroid hormone T3. Studies have shown that lower levels of selenium will affect thyroid hormone production.

First, try to integrate more selenium into your diet by consuming more of the following: Brazil nuts, tuna, beef, turkey, chicken, eggs, cottage cheese, oatmeal, rice.

Selenium is a great antioxidant when used correctly.

Dosage: 100 Micrograms daily

Vitamin A

Vitamin A appears to influence thyroid hormone receptors and it is crucial for the communication of thyroid hormones. It also acts as an antioxidant.

Sources of vitamin A include milk, eggs, liver, apricots, cantaloupe, pumpkin, squash, turnip, carrots, plums, watermelon, plantains, peas, oatmeal, broccoli, and spinach.

Dosage: 4000 International Units

Vitamin D

Vitamin D has recently been acknowledged for having over 2,000 different actions in the human body. Vitamin D helps with depression, weight loss, cancer, the immune system, and on and on and on.

It is particularly important for you because Hashimoto's is related to an immune system problem and vitamin D helps regulate the immune system.

Sources: Fish, mushrooms, eggs, meats, and fortified dairy products.

Vitamin D3 is the form of vitamin D that you want, so look for an emulsified vitamin D supplement.

Dosage: A minimum of 2,000 international units and up to 20,000. Some doctors recommend dosages of 5,000 I.U., and if you have hypothyroidism, you may need more. Opt for a vitamin D test to help with dosing.

Vitamin D testing is widely available—and I suggest you get tested because too much Vitamin D can be toxic.

I almost forgot to mention the best source of this amazing vitamin—which is the sun. However, if you're wearing clothing or sunscreen, you won't be able to produce vitamin D because it's made in the skin along with cholesterol—yes cholesterol.

I bet you thought all cholesterol was bad for you. The fact is, you need it to make hormones and, actually, vitamin D is more of a hormone than vitamin.

Zinc

Zinc helps with the production of T3, and studies have shown that when zinc levels are low so is T3 production. Research suggests that supplementation with zinc helps T3 production. Zinc also helps reduce thyroid antibodies.

Sources: Ginger, dairy, nuts, green vegetables, turkey, beef, fish, seafood, herring, and whole grains.

Dosage: 20 milligrams daily.

Progesterone

Progesterone is an estrogen and cortisol antagonist. It helps reduce excess estrogen and produce thyroid hormone—a common problem seen with hypothyroidism. You should investigate your levels of progesterone with guidance of a physician and supplement accordingly.

Vitamin E

There are many forms of Vitamin E and the most powerful form is d-alpha tocopherol. It's a great antioxidant found in green peas, spinach, asparagus, kale, cucumber, tomato, and celery. It helps against the damaging effects of polyunsaturated oils.

Vitamin E helps the body absorb iodine and helps metabolize selenium. It also helps the body convert T4 to T3.

Dosage: 400 International units daily.

Magnesium

Magnesium is a mineral that most people are deficient in and if you have hypothyroidism, you can bet your level is low. Magnesium helps prevent high blood pressure, heart disease, diabetes, and helps absorb calcium.

High levels of magnesium can be found in shrimp, clams, crab, coconut, brown rice, almonds, walnuts, peas, dried seaweed, and cocoa.

Dosage: 200 milligrams daily

Essential fatty acids

Essential fatty acids include EPA and DHA. These fats have a number of actions in the body; they help cells communicate, reduce inflammation, and produce necessary hormones.

The best sources are found in cold-water fish like mackerel, herring, sardines, and salmon.

Omega fatty acids are a very common supplement found in just about every store. However, you should know, because it's an oil, it is very sensitive to temperature change, oxygen, and sunlight exposure. If you're going to supplement with essential fatty acids, it is imperative that you find a good manufacturer that tests their product for heavy metal toxicity.

Dosage: 1,000—2,000 milligrams daily.

So, Now What?

You're probably thinking, wow, those are a lot of pills to take...

Slow down a second. There is an easy way to make sure you get what you need into your diet to help your body fight hypothyroidism and weight gain.

As you may have noticed, I have listed some foods of where you can get these nutrients...

Start with the food.

Next, you will realize that most of these nutrients can be found in a good multivitamin and multimineral supplement. Purchase a good multi and take it religiously.

Then, find the missing nutrients like fish oil and purchase it—and take it along with your multi.

Lastly, find a physician that will test you for vitamin/mineral deficiencies. This is a much better and sure-fire way of determining what supplements to take.

Remember, it's not one nutrient that is going to make or break you. Food is the most important part of this program, and supplements will help if you eat correctly.

Below you will find a list of great supplement companies. As I have said before, you get what you pay for. Don't go shopping around a discount store for medicine; the items are discounted for a reason.

At times, you may only be able to purchase some of these supplements through a licensed practitioner and for a good reason; they should be treated as medicine, not candy.

Also, this is just a small sample of what may help your condition. Depending on the cause of your hypothyroidism, you may benefit from other nutrients.

If you have questions about other nutrients that may help your condition, please contact my office.

By the way, I have no obligation or connection to any of the companies listed other than I use their products for helping my patients, family, and friends.

Resources

Books:

Encyclopedia of Natural Medicine, Murray/Pizzorno

Products and Companies:

Vitamin D — Biotics Research Corporation www.bioticsresearch.com

Essential Fatty Acids — Nordic Naturals **www.nordicnaturals.com**

Multivitamin — Nutri-Spec 800-736-4320 www.nutri-spec.net

Probiotics — Integrative Therapeutics www.integrativeinc.com

Neutraceuticals — Vital Nutrients www.vitalnutrients.net

Chapter 8
Detoxification

I'm sure you are familiar with the word detoxification and unfortunately it doesn't have a friendly connotation to it. You hear about down-and-out celebrities going through detox, or maybe you've seen actors portraying someone in movies going through this process. The sights and sounds of people experiencing a detox are not pleasant.

Most of these situations are due to someone trying to separate themselves from their dependence on a narcotic or alcohol. This form of a detox can be very dramatic, dangerous, and encouraged because of a life-threatening health condition.

However, there are many different types of detoxes and many reasons for doing them.

Recently, there has been some popularity with detoxes for weight loss. This type of detox like many others has some health benefits, risks, and drawbacks. Regardless of the reason for detoxification, its purpose is to remove toxic substances from the human body so that the body can return to homeostasis.

Homeostasis means that the body will function at a higher metabolic rate and more efficiently.

The amazing thing about the human body is that it already has built-in detoxification systems. These systems help your body detoxify harmful substances through urination, defecation, and perspiration.

The detox that will be used here is nothing more than speeding up your body's normal detoxification process by using certain supplements and removing foods and beverages that your body may be sensitive to.

You may be thinking that you probably don't eat or drink anything that is toxic or harmful to your body, but there are many things in the foods you eat and in the beverages you drink that are very stressful to your body.

Give Your Liver a Break and Lose Weight

Two common substances you may consume that put your detoxification systems in overdrive are caffeine and alcohol. Alcohol, as you may already know, is harmful to the body if consumed in large quantities and regularly.

Caffeine is a substance you may not think is harmful to the body, but there is research showing the body's heightened level of detoxification when caffeine is consumed.

Drinking caffeine will elevate certain liver enzymes in your body. This is a very similar reaction that may occur when you take over-the-counter pain medication such as Tylenol.

Some medical authorities suggest that your body will recover easily from taking non-prescription medication and it probably will. But if you do this day in and day out, the long-term side effects can be detrimental.

It's the everyday use of certain substances that can be a burden and cause harm.

When your body recognizes certain substances as synthetic and possibly harmful, it steps up its detoxification process.

I'm not suggesting that you can never drink alcohol, coffee, or take over-the-counter pain medication. But the purpose of the detox is to remove these substances from your diet for a period of time so that your body can get a break from being overstressed.

When your body is not overworked trying to remove harmful substances from its environment, it can then process foods faster and more easily.

Everyone reacts differently to substances like caffeine and alcohol—and any other food. Paying close attention to how your body feels when you consume them, especially after a detox, will tell you if you should be consuming them or not.

When you remove all these stressful substances from your diet, your body may react adversely from their removal, but the way you will feel afterward will be well worth it.

Some of the symptoms you may experience through a detox are headaches, body aches, flu-like symptoms, skin irritations, mild fever, constipation, diarrhea, and upset stomach.

The most common symptom is a mild headache and usually only lasts for a couple of days due to caffeine withdrawal.

If you are doing a detox, it is wise to consult with a medical professional experienced with the process, especially if you take prescription medication or are being treated for any health condition.

The process of going through a detoxification helps remove harmful substances that have been stored in certain tissues and organs of the body for weeks, months, and even years. Some of these substances include heavy metals, pesticides, herbicides, hormone disruptors, and certain medications.

Another reason for participating in a detox is that it gives your organs and organ systems a break from the burden of processing all the junk your body needs to get rid of. It can help your body reduce inflammation, heal your gut, help you lose weight, normalize blood sugar, reduce cholesterol, and clear up your skin.

Other Benefits from Detoxification

There are many benefits from doing a detox other than the immediate relief from certain bodily symptoms.

A detox can not only help you feel better and lose weight, but it can also help you recognize what substances or foods you consume regularly your body is sensitive or allergic to.

Most people don't realize they have a food sensitivity until they remove the food from their diet for a couple of weeks and then reintroduce that food back into their diet and observe a reaction.

This is the only true test to determining foods sensitivities and allergies. There are certain saliva and blood tests available, but not all of them are accurate.

Your body's reaction to food in a clean body is the true test.

Hypothyroidism has a number of different causes and just about any one of these can be helped through a detox.

Some causes of hypothyroidism relate to hormone imbalances where the body cannot clear certain hormones through the liver to keep your body in balance. Your liver is the main organ responsible for detoxification, and if it's rejuvenated through a detox, it will reduce your symptoms.

Another cause of hypothyroidism is from toxicity of certain heavy metals. Again, these harmful substances are cleared through the liver.

Other causes of hypothyroidism are due to stress on the body through your external environment, which causes an internal stress or disruption of certain organs and hormones.

Whatever the cause of hypothyroidism, you'll help your condition and lose weight from detoxification.

However, once you've gone through this process, do not return to your old habits.

Once you've discovered that your body doesn't like a certain food, do not go back eating this food after your detox—or you'll be back to square one.

The whole idea of doing a detox is to remove harmful substances from the body and to identify foods that your body doesn't like.

It may be tough to remove more than a couple of foods you like from your diet after you have identified that these foods are bad for you, but try to remove at least one. Then, try another detox in three months and remove another food.

Eventually, you may be able to return to eating a food that you were sensitive to in a few months, but your body needs time to heal.

However, with hypothyroidism you should never return to eating gluten.

Another great thing that happens after a detox is that you will lose your cravings for the sweet stuff.

A detox will help normalize your blood sugar, reduce the stress on your pancreas, and eventually help your body become more sensitive to insulin. The stabilization of blood sugar will eliminate your cravings as long as you stay away from highly processed sweet treats.

The Quick and Easy Detox

There are a number of different ways to help your body speed up the detoxification process. One way is by drinking more water.

Water has a number of important functions in the human body as discussed here in different chapters. And it is crucial for your body to detoxify harmful substances.

As mentioned earlier—your body rids itself of harmful substances through perspiration, urination, and defecation. So, when you're going through a detox your body is trying to remove more than its normal share of bad stuff. You'll need more water than what you usually drink to help flush toxins out of your body.

You should drink plenty of room-temperature purified water throughout the day when going through this process. You can squeeze a lemon or lime wedge into the water for taste and to help alkalize the body.

Other beverages permitted during a detox include herbal tea, green tea, and vegetable juices.

Another great way to get the impurities out of your body is through sweating.

Now, I'm not suggesting you run ten miles when trying to detox. In fact, you may not feel like exercising at all during this time; but if you have the energy to work out, light workouts will help you sweat and aid in the removal of toxins.

You can go to your local health club or spa and use the steam room. This will open up your pores and help you sweat more without exercising to remove the bad stuff.

But don't try lounging in a hot steam room for too long. It's better to steam at lower temperatures for a longer time than to use a really hot steam room. There are dangers of steaming too long in super-hot rooms, so be careful.

Dry saunas are another great way to detoxify the body from harmful substances. The great news is now even people with heart conditions who should not use high temperatures for detoxification can detox with far Infrared Saunas. These use special technology without all the high heat.

Pop a Pill and Detox

There is one extra step you can do to help your body remove the excess garbage that's been tied up inside of you—which is taking a supplement or two.

I am a big proponent of supplementation, but you do have to make the necessary changes in your diet first before taking a supplement because no supplement is going to work magic all by itself. Supplements cannot overcome all the nasty things you may be putting into your body.

Also, it makes a big difference where you buy your supplements from and who makes them. Picking up a couple of bottles of natural supplements at your local store without any knowledge about them will leave you disappointed in the results.

First, do research on whatever it is you're looking for; this way you'll know the active ingredients and can find it when you turn the bottle over.

A lot of companies will add binders, fillers, and other unnecessary ingredients that you don't need. Some companies may not test their supplements, nor do they care where they get their raw materials from. Some companies buy other companies' supplements and just put their name on them.

Take some time and call the company and ask questions like: where do you get your raw materials from, are your products third party tested, what is the efficacy of product X, do you offer refunds?

Questions like these help you separate good supplement companies from bad ones.

However, if you want the best companies, look to your local natural healthcare practitioner or nutritionist. Some of the best companies restrict their product sales only to healthcare practitioners. They back up their products because they rely on repeat sales from multiple products for treating different conditions. Basically, they're selling medicine and if it doesn't work, the doctor will know and the company won't make money.

Buying supplements through a practitioner may be more costly, but remember the old saying, "You get what you pay for."

The Best Supplements for Detox

There will be recommendations for products and companies in the resource section.

Now that you know a bit about how to get your hands on a good supplement—the supplement you want to take during this detox is called milk thistle.

Milk thistle's formal name is *silybum marianum*. Milk thistle will help reduce inflammation of the liver, protect the liver, and aid it during detoxification.

Your liver is one of the main organs through which all chemicals in your body are detoxified. Taking this supplement will greatly improve the results of your detox—assuming you are following the diet plan.

Just follow the instructions on the bottle you purchase to help you with dosing.

Another great supplement that helps up-regulate your immune system and helps with detoxification elimination is a **probiotic.**

Did you know that you have more bacteria in your intestinal tract than cells in your entire body?

Your intestines are loaded with bacteria, some good and some bad. When the bad bacteria outnumber the good bacteria, it leads to a health condition called dysbiosis. And dysbiosis can lead to other health problems.

One of the jobs of the good bacteria is to neutralize foreign invaders that get into your gut. In other words, the good bacteria represent your immune system.

I bet that you didn't know your immune system starts in your gut.

Adding a probiotic to your program helps with digestion, absorption, constipation, elimination, and your immune system.

There are a lot of probiotic products on the market, and once again what you buy and where you buy it from makes a huge difference.

Another great resource for health products is your local health food store. Most towns have one and I am not talking about the big chain stores. Find a small independent health food store and get to know the owner. They are probably very educated on what works and what doesn't.

Most of the stores will have a refrigerated section with probiotics. Not all need to be refrigerated, but this is a good place to start. Look for products that contain *Lactobacillus acidophilus and Bifidobacterium.* The supplement should have a minimum of 1 billion CFU. It will state this on the back of the supplement. Follow the directions of the manufacturer.

Also, it is wise to supplement your diet and detox program with a good multivitamin/multimineral and some additional antioxidants.

Vitamin C is a great water-soluble antioxidant that helps with detoxification along with neutralizing free radicals. It has many other functions in the body, such as building connective tissue and supporting various organs like your adrenal glands. It is a cheap and wise investment for regular use.

The supplements recommended are a good starting point for a detoxification program. There are other forms of detoxes that require multiple supplements and shakes—and they can be very good and costly. Check with your local Naprapath, Naturopath, Chiropractor, and nutritionist if you're interested in taking the extra step. But remember, your main focus is what you will be eating and drinking.

If you are interested in a more complete detoxification program with guidance, you can also call my office for support.

Detox On the Run

Now that you know what you can do to help detoxify your body, I will help you put it all together.

There are a lot of detoxification plans and diets available on the market. Some are complicated and require a lot of work and fasting, while others may use a lot of supplements and certain procedures like enemas.

Some detoxes require you to only drink water, others to drink just vegetable juices, and there are detoxes that suggest you should use ionizing footbaths.

Some of these techniques do work; some are dangerous, and some are unnecessary.

This detox program is designed to identify food allergies/sensitivities, give your body a break from the Standard American Diet, normalize blood sugar, and remove some of the toxins that may be causing you harm.

I realize you still have to go to work and you have obligations that you cannot put on hold.

In a perfect world, you would do a detox at a beautiful resort and spa on a vacation weekend in the Bahamas. But this is the real world, and I have designed it for real people like you.

So, you will be able to eat and drink and go about your normal everyday life without putting things on hold. However, there may be times during the first couple of days when you will want to limit your daily activities.

Detoxification Diet Basics

Foods to Avoid

All gluten-containing foods like wheat, rye, oats, and barley, which are commonly found in breads, pasta, and other products made from refined flour.

The most common food allergies are from this group of foods. Avoiding these foods for a couple of weeks will allow your body to relax and clear itself out. You may not even know you have an allergy to these foods because the symptoms are so subtle.

Alcohol, caffeine (coffee, black teas, sodas), fruit juice, and soy milk.

Alcohol and caffeine are very hard on your liver, so give it a vacation!

Pork, cold cuts, bacon, hot dogs, canned meat, sausage, and shellfish.

These meats are highly processed and may contain fillers, antibiotics, estrogens, nitrates, msg and other binders and/or natural flavorings.

All dairy (milk, cheese, yogurt, butter, etc.)

Dairy food allergies are very common. Stay away from creamy salad dressings (ranch, garlic) as they may contain dairy.

Foods high in fats and oils, including peanuts, margarine, shortening, and other refined oils.

Most oils are highly processed and should be avoided to lessen the burden on your body. They may cause a disruption in hormones.

Fruit of any kind

Fruit is very high in sugar and will make it harder to lose weight. Also, sugar causes an elevation of certain hormones which stress certain organs.

Other

Any other foods that you're aware of that cause your body to react adversely.

Shopping List

Vegetables Asparagus, avocado, bell peppers, zucchini, yams, yellow wax beans, peas, parsley, bok choy, Swiss chard, shallots, leaks, green beans, okra, squash, chives, mushrooms, cucumber, sweet potato, pinto beans, spinach, mixed greens, red-leaf or romaine lettuce, stir fry veggies, carrots, celery, eggplant, pea pods, kale, and beets.

Choose organic and local if possible.

Meat/seafood choices Chicken breast, turkey breast, flank steak, lamb chops, duck, Cornish game hen, flounder, salmon, halibut, haddock, cod, red snapper, orange roughy, tilapia, perch, anchovies, herring, sardines, pollock, and mackerel.

Choose organic, grass fed, and wild meats and seafood. Avoid tuna because of high mercury content. Also, avoid shellfish such as mussels, shrimp, lobster, scallops.

Eggs   *Preferably cage-free, hormone free, omega 3, and organic*

Grains   Cream of rice, millet, white rice (not minute), tapioca, quinoa, 100% buckwheat, and amaranth.

Drinks   Herbal tea, green tea, non-fluorinated, non-chlorinated water.

Dressings Organic extra virgin olive oil, citrus (lemon, lime), basil, oregano.

Misc.   Raw almonds, rice crackers, almond butter.

Sample Detox Diet

Day 1

Breakfast: 1 cup plain goat milk yogurt, cinnamon, chopped almonds and stevia to taste.

Lunch: Spinach salad and sliced mushrooms, extra virgin olive oil and lemon juice with baked chicken breast or fish.

Dinner: Baked turkey breast with 1/4 sweet potato and steamed asparagus or green beans.

Day 2

Breakfast: 1 slice of rice bread with organic sugar-free almond butter and raw celery or cucumber.

Lunch: Fish tacos (not breaded) with onions, cilantro, tomato, sliced avocado, fresh lime juice on 1 corn tortilla.

Dinner: Stir fry pork and veggies over 1/4 cup of white rice. Optional mixed green salad with extra virgin olive oil and citrus.

Day 3

Breakfast: Two-egg veggie omelet with avocado.

Lunch: Buffalo burger (no bread) topped with lettuce, tomato, pickles, Dijon and 2/3 cup lentil soup or split pea.

Dinner: Chicken baked with lemon, olive oil, and oregano. Serve over 1 cup of spaghetti squash with asparagus spears and sun-dried tomatoes.

Day 4

Breakfast: Nitrate-free turkey or chicken sausage with 1/4 cup roasted sweet potato.

Lunch: Mexican salad with seasoned ground sirloin, lettuce, 1/3 cup kidney beans, fresh salsa, guacamole.

Dinner: Halibut or cod fillet with steamed spinach.

Day 5

Breakfast: Salmon with sliced cucumber, dill, and goat cheese.

Lunch: Grilled chicken breast over a bed of romaine with avocado, tomato, cucumber, and extra virgin olive oil and lemon juice.

Dinner: Steak with onions, peppers, and mushrooms, 1/4 sweet potato and grilled zucchini.

Day 6

Breakfast: Two soft-boiled eggs and asparagus spears.

Lunch: Stir fry veggies, 1/4 cup white rice, and two small lamb chops.

Dinner: Turkey burger patty, steamed green beans, and 1/4 cup baked sweet potato fries.

Day 7

Breakfast: Crumbled nitrate-free turkey sausage sautéed with onions, mushrooms, and peppers on 1 small corn tortilla.

Lunch: Almonds, goat cheese, and sun dried tomatoes over a bead of romaine with steak and extra virgin olive oil.

Dinner: Baked salmon over 1/4 cup of white rice with steamed yellow squash and zucchini.

How to Get Started?

The above food menu is just an example of how to eat, not necessarily what to eat...

If you don't like the food in the menu—change it. There is nothing worse than trying to stick to a diet of food that you don't like—and that's one reason for failure with diets.

One way to guarantee success with a new food program is to design it yourself with foods you enjoy and that you know you'll eat.

So, start preparing by going through the example food lists for shopping and start pairing up proteins and veggies. Make an example menu for two weeks. You can always make changes as you go; and if it's written down, it will be easier to stick to.

Once you have your foods—start cooking. You can prepare a couple of meals ahead of time, you can even cook for the whole week in one day and then just freeze your meals.

The nice thing about these meals is they're simple. Most meals are composed of a protein and some veggies—both of which are quick and easy to cook. Some organic veggies are sold precooked and all you have to do is defrost them by letting them sit out at room temperature.

This is very convenient for work. Just place some veggies in tupperware and drizzle with olive oil and Celtic sea salt. If you do this first thing in the morning, by the time lunch rolls around the veggies will be ready to eat.

Another great suggestion is to prepare meals the night before work, otherwise you might not make the time in the morning and then you'll end up eating something convenient that you will regret later.

If you ever have a doubt about what to eat, always remember—stick to the list, at least for the first two weeks. The first two weeks are crucial to your success. Remember, it's just two weeks.

After the first two weeks, you'll be allowed to add additional food into your meal plan.

What If I'm a Vegetarian?

If you're a vegetarian, this could be easier or harder for you, depending on your habits.

Some vegetarians eat lots of veggies, but they also eat a lot of carbs from processed convenient foods or other food made with artificial meat from soy, and these foods are NOT on the list.

Unfortunately, if you eat dairy and you're a vegetarian, you still should avoid it for a couple of weeks to determine if you have a sensitivity to casein or lactose.

You can replace cow's milk products with sheep, goat, or buffalo products. Also, you can get cheese products made from rice. Or you can use organic fermented soy products such as tofu. Either substitute will work, just make sure you eat protein with every meal.

If you choose animal products other than cow's milk, just make sure you read the ingredient label because some manufacturers may add casein.

How Much Is Too Much?

Just a word about serving sizes...

Your protein should be at least three ounces in weight or the size of the palm of your hand. You don't need more than this, but if you wish to eat an extra half of serving, it will not harm you, just try not to make this a habit.

When it comes to veggies, eat as much as you want with the exception of starchy veggies like potatoes, corn, peas, and carrots.

If you get hungry in between meals, feel free to snack on veggies, raw almonds, and rice crackers with almond butter. Try to limit almonds to a 1/4 cup, and rice crackers with nut butter to 6-8 crackers.

Checklist

- There are certain rules that you must follow when on this program.
- Don't stray away from the list.
- You must eat breakfast—it's the most important meal!
- You must eat three square meals a day.
- Every meal should have protein, fat, and carbohydrate (carbs from veggies).
- Try to rotate meals so you aren't eating the same meal every day.
- Never eat gluten or casein (the protein found in cow's milk; other animal milk is ok).
- Drink lots of water between meals.

Resources

Books:

The Liver Cleansing Diet, Sandra Cabot, MD

The Master Cleanse, Stanley Buroughs

Medical Detoxification programs:

Biotics Research, www.bioticsresearch.com

Apex Energetics, www.orderapex.com

Chapter 9

The Meal Plan

Hopefully, you've been through the detox part of this program and you're feeling better.

The detoxification segment is very important, so don't skip it.

Remember, this is a <u>program,</u> not just a diet—and you have medical needs, opposed to someone who just wants to lose a few pounds. Stick with the program and you'll be successful.

By now, you should have more energy, less digestive upsets and constipation, and you should be a couple of pounds lighter.

By the way, I should point out that, when it comes to weight loss, an ideal amount of weight to lose is .5–2 pounds per week.

I know you've probably seen contestants on The Biggest Loser lose 10–15 pounds per week, but one thing you don't know is the content of the weight they lose.

When someone loses more than 3 pounds per week, generally it is from muscle and water loss—not fat.

It is extremely hard to lose large amounts of body fat in one week. This is why I suggest a lower number, it's more realistic and a number of pounds you can consistently lose without being disappointed week after week.

If you follow a low calorie diet without a consideration for how much fat and protein you eat along with an improper exercise program, you can lose one of the most important metabolic components you have—MUSCLE.

So don't be disappointed if you haven't lost a large amount of weight—be patient. Remember, your body has been stuck in a rut for a while, and it takes time to kick-start your thyroid.

Also, I have worked with patients before who only lost five pounds, yet they lost two inches off their waist. Which would you rather have—a smaller waist or a smaller number on the scale?

The next step in this process is to evaluate if you have an allergy/sensitivity to dairy products.

Dairy products can be very nutritious if you can get them from a raw organic source.

Dairy is a very common allergy just like gluten, but there is no connection between dairy allergies and hypothyroidism.

But if you do have a problem with dairy, it can cause an immune response and make it harder for you to lose weight and cause other symptoms.

The object in the next week of the food plan following the two-week detox is to determine if you have a sensitivity to dairy.

Does Dairy Work for Me?

Ok, it's test time. After your two weeks of detoxification, your immune system should have settled down, your blood sugar should be stable, and you're ready for the next step.

Now you are going to test your body to see if you can tolerate dairy products by adding one source of dairy back into your diet on the first day after the detox.

Don't add more than one dairy food back into your diet on this day. Also, you will not eat any more dairy products for the next couple of days.

As a rule, never test more than one food group every couple of days, because your body can have a delayed reaction from a food up to 72 hours later.

However, most food reactions will occur within a few hours after eating a food your body is sensitive to.

Here's what to look for:

Immediately following breakfast, start paying attention to how you feel...

Signs and symptoms of food allergies/sensitivities include:

- belching
- bloating
- gas
- upset stomach
- headache
- diarrhea
- constipation
- coughing
- excessive phlegm
- itchy skin
- watery or itchy eyes
- confusion
- light headedness
- brain fog
- short attention span
- forgetfulness
- irritability
- anxious feeling
- nervousness
- lethargy

The symptoms can vary, but don't be confused about these symptoms compared to how you normally feel.

Just think about how you have felt after your last couple of meals and compare that to any of the symptoms listed above.

If you experience any of these symptoms or you just don't feel right after you eat dairy, chances are your body is sensitive to this food.

This doesn't mean you can never eat dairy again. All this means is that you will have to eliminate dairy products for the next three months.

Following twelve weeks off dairy, try reintroducing dairy products into your diet again to see if your immune system has calmed down.

If you don't have a reaction to eating dairy on day one of this meal plan, you can continue eating it every other day for the first week.

If you still have no reaction after the first week, then dairy can be added to your daily menu.

Snacks

At this point, you should still try to keep sugar out of your diet until the fourth week. This includes alcohol, coffee, fruit, and most grains.

If you do get hungry, you can allow yourself a snack. Here are some great snack ideas that will leave you satisfied, help with your blood sugar, hormones, and cravings.

- Low sodium beef jerky
- Almonds
- Pecans
- Walnuts
- Unsalted sunflower seeds
- Unsalted pumpkin seeds
- Hard-boiled egg
- Cheese stick
- Avocado or tomato slices
- Raw vegetables: celery, cherry tomatoes, cucumbers, mushrooms with salsa, guacamole, or humus.
- Shrimp
- Roll-ups with meat/cheese
- Slices of left-over chicken or beef

Try to keep the serving of nuts/seeds to 1/4 cup.

Dressings and Other Condiments

In order to turn the corner with your health and body weight, you will have to consume foods that are homemade, including your dressings.

This is a lot easier than you think and they taste much better.

Start with cold-pressed organic extra virgin olive oil. Add fresh lemon or lime juice instead of vinegar to make a salad dressing. Use two part olive oil to one part lemon.

Vinegar is one condiment that can raise your blood sugar if you have too much of it. Ketchup and mustard can do the same.

You can add sea salt, pepper, and some herbs to your dressing, such as parsley for flavoring.

Preparing your own dressings helps cut out sugar and bad oils which may disrupt your hormones.

You can also cut out sugar by using spices and dry rubs on your meats instead of ketchup and barbeque sauce.

This way, you'll get the health benefits of the herbs and reduce your sugar intake.

Instead of using mayonnaise for salads and sandwiches, you can use plain yogurt with lemon juice and a bit of salt or try using humus. You can now get humus in a variety of flavors.

Just use your imagination when it comes to dressing-up salads, veggies, and other foods.

The main idea is to get away from commercial made products and to get you back into the kitchen.

If you do buy commercial products, buy organic products from smaller companies. Trader Joe's is a great example of where to buy these products, or try your local health food store.

Meal Plan Week One

Day 1

Breakfast: 1/2 cup of organic whole milk cottage cheese with sliced cucumber and celery.

Lunch: Grecian chicken with a small Greek salad with onions, tomatoes, feta cheese, cucumbers, and olive oil/citrus dressing.

Dinner: Baked halibut with 1/4 cup of white rice and grilled eggplant.

Day 2

Breakfast: Scrambled eggs with mushrooms, onions, and green peppers.

Lunch: A bowl of chili made with ground beef or turkey, onions, peppers, tomatoes, and kidney beans.

Dinner: Carne asada with a side of black beans and julienned zucchini and yellow squash.

Day 3

Breakfast: Organic goat milk yogurt with pecans, cinnamon, and stevia.

Lunch: Two small lettuce wraps with turkey and provolone and 1 cup of vegetable soup.

Dinner: Baked salmon with asparagus and 1/3 cup of chick peas.

Day 4

Breakfast: Breakfast burrito with scrambled eggs, salsa, and avocado on one small corn tortilla.

Lunch: One hamburger patty with a 1/4 cup of baked sweet potato fries and a small garden salad.

Dinner: Chicken breast with BBQ rub and a 1/2 cup of black beans and corn.

Day 5

Breakfast: Chicken or turkey sausage with avocado and tomatoes slices.

Lunch: Three bean salad with left-over chicken breast slices.

Dinner: Two shrimp kabobs with onion, peppers, and mushrooms.

Day 6

Breakfast: 1/2 cup organic whole milk cottage cheese with cucumber and celery slices.

Lunch: Fish tacos with salsa and guacamole on corn tortilla.

Dinner: A bowl of 12 bean soup with chicken and turkey sausage.

Day 7

Breakfast: Two-egg omelet with spinach, tomatoes, and mushrooms.

Lunch: Tuna or salmon salad lettuce wraps with a cup of veggie soup.

Dinner: Chicken quesadillas with salsa, avocado, and a side of black beans.

The Next Step...

At this point, if you have no problems with eating dairy products, then it's something you can put back on your menu.

There is one particular form of dairy that contains a wide variety of amino acids, it's a great source of protein and you can eat for breakfast or as a meal replacement.

What I'm referring to is whey protein.

Whey is great for making smoothies for breakfast or as a post-workout meal.

But remember, you must treat a smoothie as a meal—meaning it should contain protein, fat, and a carbohydrate and not too many carbs.

The problem with commercial smoothies and the way most people make them is that they're *loaded* with sugar.

Most smoothies contain fruit juice, fruit concentrate, and real fruit, but not much of anything else. In fact, I've seen some commercial smoothie franchises add sherbet ice cream to their smoothies. Also, some smoothies can be in excess of 500 calories.

So, what happens after drinking this type of smoothie? Your blood sugar will sky-rocket.

This is NOT what you want.

A smoothie is supposed to be a quick healthy meal replacement option, but if you're just adding sugar without protein and fat, it's just a sweet drink, isn't it?

You can still create a great tasting smoothie without sabotaging your weight loss program.

Here's how...

Smoothies

Start with a couple of scoops of a good whey protein, add some liquid to the whey such as almond milk, rice milk, coconut milk, or water. One half of a cup of liquid is plenty, but don't add fruit juice!

Next, add fruit.

Some of the best fruits for smoothies are berries; blueberries, blackberries, raspberries, strawberries. However, strawberries are considered a goitrogen, so use them sparingly.

One-third to one-half of a cup of berries works well. I think frozen berries work better than fresh berries for smoothies.

I use a combination of a banana and some berries. Bananas are great for adding body and texture to the smoothie, but they are high in sugar. So, use only half of a banana and use bananas that are green tipped.

The longer a banana ages, the browner it gets and the more sugar it will contain.

The next component that needs to be added is fat.

If you're using almond milk or coconut milk, you're getting some fat into the smoothie—but not enough. So, add one teaspoon of coconut oil to your smoothie.

Remember, coconut oil is very metabolic and you should be getting two teaspoons of it into your diet daily.

Another consideration for your smoothies is vegetables. Vegetables can add a lot of nutrients to your drink and you can get 2-3 servings of veggies in one meal.

Some veggies to consider are spinach, celery, cucumbers, grasses, and beats—just beware of the goitrogens.

One of the easiest ways to include organic veggies into your smoothie is to buy a powered mix of dried ground-up vegetables or greens.

Blend and enjoy!

It may take some trial and error to find a combination of taste and texture that you like, but try to include smoothies into your diet because they can be very nutritious.

Fruit and Grains

The fourth week of this program is the turning point and the time when you can start adding some fruit and grains back into your diet.

By now, your blood sugar and related hormones should have normalized, and your body should be functioning more efficiently.

However, you don't want to overdo it! You can add small portions of fruit to your meals without having an adverse reaction.

Always remember that you shouldn't eat fruit by itself for the sake of trying to keep your blood sugar stable. For instance, if you're going to snack on an apple—have some cheese with it.

The fruits you will be eating will come from a category of low sugar fruits with lots of nutrients like berries.

The complex carbohydrates that you will be allowed to eat will be non-gluten forms of carbs that are non reactive and very safe to eat, like rice.

The key to eating carbohydrates like grains, pastas, and rice is to keep the portions small. They should never be the focus of any meal. Think of them like a small side dish—1/4 - 1/3 of a cup.

Your meal should be composed of a protein, fat, and vegetable—both raw and cooked, and a small portion of complex carbohydrate like rice.

In an ideal world, you would get your carbohydrates from vegetables and some fruits. If you can follow this suggestion, you will not have many difficulties with your blood sugar, energy levels, or body weight.

Also, if you need to eat complex carbohydrates, try to limit your servings to just one meal in the day. This way, you get something to look forward to and you will not abuse them.

Fruits

Fresh or frozen organic berries
- Raspberries
- Blackberries
- Boysenberries
- Cranberries
- Blueberries

Fresh organic apples
- Granny Smith
- Red delicious

Citrus
- Lemon
- Lime
- Grapefruit

Grains

Non-gluten breads, pastas, crackers
- Amaranth
- Buckwheat/groats/kasha
- Cassava (arrowroot)
- Chickpea (garbanzo)
- Job's Tears
- Millet
- Montina
- Oats, but oats can be contaminated with wheat and other grains.
- Quinoa
- Ragi
- Rice
- Sorghum
- Tapioca
- Taro root
- Teff

Meal Plan Week Two

Day 1

Breakfast: Whey protein smoothie with 1/2 banana, 1/4 cup blueberries, 4-6 oz. non-sweetened rice or almond milk, and 1 tsp. coconut oil.

Lunch: Grilled chicken breast with sautéed spinach, mushrooms, and lemon juice.

Dinner: Baked salmon, asparagus, and 1/3 cup of wild rice.

Day 2

Breakfast: Two poached eggs and one slice of gluten-free bread lightly buttered.

Lunch: Two lettuce wraps with turkey, provolone, avocado, tomato, alfalfa sprouts, and humus. Four rice crackers with almond butter.

Dinner: 6 oz. petite beef filet, asparagus spears, 1/3 sweet potato.

Day 3

Breakfast: 2/3 cup of organic whole cow's milk yogurt and 1/3 cup mixed berries.

Lunch: Baked cod, 1/3 cup of brown rice, and small side salad.

Dinner: Vegetable beef soup with a side of buffalo mozzarella, tomatoes, and basil.

Day 4

Breakfast: Whey protein smoothie with 4-6 oz. of non-sweetened rice/almond milk, 1/2 banana, 1/4 of berries, and 1 tsp. of coconut oil.

Lunch: One hamburger patty with a 1/3 cup of baked sweet potato fries.

Dinner: Two chicken tacos on a lettuce wrap with salsa, guacamole, side of black beans.

Day 5

Breakfast: One veggie omelet.

Lunch: Chicken Cesar salad with homemade dressing and a cup of veggie soup.

Dinner: Pork tenderloin, collard greens, and 1/3 cup of wild rice.

Day 6

Breakfast: 1.5 slices of gluten-free bread and almond butter.

Lunch: BBQ chicken with homemade rub and a side of green beans, and black beans.

Dinner: Gluten-free pita with onions, zucchini, yellow squash, feta cheese, and hummus.

Day 7

Breakfast: 1/2 cup of organic whole milk cottage cheese and 1/2 of an apple.

Lunch: Cob salad with turkey, cheese, avocado, turkey bacon, with homemade dressing.

Dinner: Skirt steak strips, pea pods, sprouts, mushrooms over 1/3 cup of rice.

You may look at this meal plan and think that you don't like these foods, or you can't eat certain foods, or how can this meal plan really help?

Well, as you can see, there's no magic food in the meal plan that's going to turn you into a Greek god/goddess overnight.

But what you may not see is everything that I've been talking about since the start of this program.

There are no fake foods in the meal plan.

There is no boxed, bagged, or canned food.

There are no processed foods.

There is very little sugar in the plan.

The meals are balanced.

The meals contain foods from nature.

There are no food colorings.

There are no preservatives.

You don't have to eat these exact foods, but you should follow these guidelines.

10,000 years ago, there was no such thing as grains. People ate wild animals, nuts, seeds, berries, and veggies.

Your body is not much different now than it was 10,000 years ago, but your diet is much, much different.

I'm not suggesting you eat like a caveman—though some would make this suggestion.

The magic is not in the meal plan, but in how you recondition your body by the removing the foods that your body doesn't like or need and replacing them with wholesome natural foods.

When you take the garbage out of your diet and keep it out, when you let your body heal and detox and add nutrient dense food, it can be like flipping on a metabolic switch.

This is how you lose weight, gain energy, and rebuild your body so it functions better.

Checklist

- Each meal should contain macronutrients that build hormones—FAT.
- Each meal should contain macronutrients that build body tissue—PROTEIN.
- Each meal should contain macronutrients that produce energy—CARBS.
- Each meal should contain natural sources of macronutrients—NOT MAN-MADE.
- Each meal should be balanced and NOT dominated by carbohydrates.

Resources

Books:

Nutrition and Physical Degeneration, Weston A. Price, D.D.S.

Nourishing Traditions, Sally Fallon

The Metabolic Typing Diet, William Wolcott

Websites:

www.GlutenFreeWorks.com

www.Coconutoil.com

www.Mercola.com

www.Grasslandbeef.com

www.PamKilleen.com

www.DyingToLookGood.com

www.WestonAPrice.org

www.NancyAppleton.com

www.ppnf.org

www.DoctorYourself.com

www.TheFactsAboutFitness.com

www.Distance-Healer.com

www.RealMilk.com

Chapter 10

The Exercise Guide for Hypothyroidism

One the biggest contributing factors to hypothyroidism is stress, and you can greatly improve your symptoms by reducing stress on the body.

But guess what...

Exercise is a form of stress, and if you have hypothyroidism, you should be very careful how much you exercise.

There are many people who exercise without caution and to an extreme. In such cases, the body can actually resist weight loss because of overuse. Here's why...

When under stress, the body produces a number of hormones one of which is cortisol.

Cortisol has a number of actions in the body, and when you're constantly under stress cortisol levels will remain high and this will make losing body fat difficult.

If you combine long, hard exercise sessions with your everyday stress, it can result in a constant flow of high cortisol in your body.

This also puts stress on the glands that produce cortisol—the adrenal glands.

One of cortisol's responsibilities is to help produce fuel when the body needs it. It does this indirectly by raising your blood sugar via the liver, brain, and muscle tissue.

In order for the body to tap into its vital reserves of energy, the body must store it for that rainy day and emergencies. And there is no better storage form of energy than FAT.

When your body is constantly under stress, it will be harder for you to lose body fat because your body's instinct is to store fat not burn it.

How you approach exercise with hypothyroidism is a sensitive balancing act, and the wrong approach can make your condition worse.

When in doubt, always remember less is more and that your body needs a break from time to time, so don't overdo it.

The next few pages will lay out a plan to ensure weight loss results even if you have a thyroid problem.

Four Big Mistakes Made With Exercise When Trying to Lose Weight

The best way to lose weight with exercise is to create a consistent exercise program with frequent sessions of exercise in short duration and high intensity.

Also, your program should include both forms of exercise cardiovascular and resistance training.

This report will cover some of the common pitfalls made with exercise when trying to lose weight.

FITT

Four of the most common mistakes made with exercise when trying to lose weight are Frequency, Intensity, Time, and Type of exercise.

To keep it simple, just remember FITT. The FITT principle stands for Frequency, Intensity, Time, and Type.

Frequency—How often you exercise

Intensity—How hard you exercise

Time—How long you exercise

Type—The type of exercise you choose

The Biggest Mistake People Make with Exercise...

In my experience, most people with weight issues don't exercise enough. In fact, how often someone exercises is the biggest mistake to avoid when trying to lose weight with exercise.

Think about it... even if you don't do the right exercises, or don't exercise long enough or if the exercise is not intense, you will still get some results as long as you're exercising.

Once, twice, or even three times a week is just not enough to lose a significant amount of weight or to transform your body.

My suggestion is to make exercise part of your life like brushing your teeth.

Make sure you do something—some form of movement at least four to six days a week. It's always good to have one day that you don't feel obligated to exercise.

However, on the seventh day, if you still want to exercise, go for a walk, stretch, or meditate do something completely different and mild compared to your normal routine.

Frequency is the biggest mistake made and for a good reason, people don't like to exercise and most hate it.

So how do you ensure that you'll do it regularly? Well, I have a few suggestions for you...

To ensure you stick to a regular exercise program, you need to schedule it. Put it on your calendar throughout the week and try to do it at the same time and place—this will create consistency and habit.

Also, you will always come up with a reason or excuse not to exercise. So the best way to make sure you'll exercise is to set up one or more condition(s) which will almost guarantee you'll do it.

For example, if you use the local gym, make an appointment with a friend to pick you up at a specific time and day. This almost guarantees you'll make it to the gym.

One of the best ways to ensure you're going to exercise is to set an appointment with a personal trainer that will charge you a fee if you don't make it.

You can also pack your gym bag the night before and set it out so you see it first thing in the morning.

Spend some time thinking about what conditions you can set up that will almost guarantee you'll exercise.

If You Fail To Do This...Your Result Will Disappoint You

One misnomer about exercise is that you must exercise for a long time to burn calories and lose weight. This is simply not true.

The most important part of exercise is that you do it frequently, which we have talked about, and the second most important part of the FITT principle is Intensity.

It's very common for people to exercise regularly throughout the week month after month without results. Why?

Well, if it's not because of their diet, it is usually because of the lack of intensity with exercise. Most people simply don't exercise at a high enough intensity to cause physical change.

The nice thing about exercise is you don't have to exercise for a long time. In fact, I discourage long sessions, but the exercise must be intense.

You can get better results from a 20-minute exercise session than from a 40-minute jog/walk as long as the intensity during the 20 minutes is high.

If you're not getting results from your workouts and you're exercising 4-6 times a week, chances are your sessions are not intense enough.

In order for you to physically change the appearance of your body, you must be willing to get out of your comfort zone—this means pushing yourself even when you don't want to. The more you do this, the better your results.

So, you may be asking yourself, how do I know if I'm exercising at a high intensity?

There are a couple of ways of determining the intensity level of exercise. One predictable way of determining how hard you are working is to use the Borg rating of perceived exertion scale or RPE.

This scale will help you equate how intense your exercise is to a particular number. This scale is based on the physical sensations a person experiences during exercise.

For example, when you exercise your heart rate will increase along with your respiration rate. You will sweat more and muscle fatigue will set in.

Familiarize yourself with the Borg RPE scale below prior to the start of a program.

Let's put some numbers to work and give you some specific examples.

6. No exertion at all
7. Extremely light
8.
9. Very Light
10.
11. Light
12.
13. Somewhat hard
14.
15. Hard (heavy)
16.
17. Very hard
18.
19. Extremely hard
20. Maximal exertion

Your goal is to exercise in a zone of 15-19. If you're just starting out, slowly work your way up to this level. In between exercises, your intensity should be a number six.

But remember, these numbers are subjective; just be honest with yourself.

How Long Do You Need to Exercise?

The third biggest mistake made with exercise when trying to lose weight relates to the length of your exercise sessions or Time.

Again, you don't need to exercise for a long time as long as your session is intense.

So how long is long enough? Well, believe it or not, there is a cardiovascular program developed by a Japanese physician that gets great results in just 4 minutes.

I know, you are probably thinking this is impossible, but it's true, there's research to support the claims.

The key, however, is intensity. Are you catching on? Here's the program...

It's best to run or use a bike for this program.

Start by warming up with 2-5 minutes of moderate exercise prior to the program; follow this by 4 minutes of intervals, and, finally, 2-5 minutes of moderate exercise to cool down after the intervals.

This program is an interval workout of 20 seconds of all-out intensity followed by 10 seconds of rest. So for 20 seconds, go as hard and as fast as you can move your body, then take 10 seconds to rest. Do this for 4 minutes and you're done!

Now, I am not suggesting that you start with this program if you're not currently exercising. You may want to start with cycles of 30 seconds of intense exercise, followed by a minute of rest. Then progress to 30 seconds on and 30 seconds off, until you're ready for the regular program.

You may be wondering why I am suggesting high intense workouts after I mentioned that too much stress for someone who has hypothyroidism is not good...

Well, it's not the stress on the body that does damage—stress is actually good for you, but it's the constant load of stress with no relief that causes problems.

In today's world, we're constantly under stress from work, family, money, time constraints, and on and on and on...

The problem is your body doesn't know the difference between physical and mental stress—your body reacts the same way. This constant load of mental, emotional, and physical stress is what overloads the body to the point of exhaustion.

This eventually leads to symptoms, conditions, and disease such as hypothyroidism.

Exercise is not bad for you as long as you limit how long you stress the body and allow it regular rest and recovery periods. This is why your program should be designed with intervals of hard work and frequent periods of rest.

Also, every session you complete should be no more than 30 minutes in length and that includes the warm-up, cool-down and rest periods.

So really, you're never exercising more than 20 minutes in one session opposed to exercising for 50-60 minutes. Exercising too long and too hard will eventually wear your body down.

You can run five miles a day and lose weight, but in the meantime you'll tear down muscle from the long stressful workouts. This will eventually lead to a plateau in weight loss because your body will eventually slow its metabolic rate due to the stress.

Muscle is the most important thing to build and maintain because it's responsible for your metabolic rate. The more muscle you have, the higher your metabolism, plain and simple.

Remember, less is more.

The latest research supports short interval sessions of high intensity for weight loss and health benefits as opposed to long steady sessions of moderate to high intense exercise.

This same concept should be applied to your weight training sessions as well. For example, exercise very hard for 30 seconds performing push-ups, then rest for one minute or 30 seconds, depending on your conditioning level.

Limit your session to 30 minutes including your warm-up and cool-down.

What Exercises Work Best?

This leads us to the last of big mistakes people make with exercise when trying to lose weight which is the Type of exercise used.

If I could suggest only one type of exercise for weight loss, it would be resistance training/lifting weights.

Why? Because there is no reason to have a separate exercise just to benefit the cardiovascular system.

You have probably tried biking, jogging, or using the elliptical to exercise, but I will tell you it's unnecessary. It's unnecessary because you can lift weights and get a cardiovascular workout along with building muscle.

Resistance training puts a high demand on your body and, as a result, there is a higher demand for blood and oxygen. This causes your heart rate and respiration rate to go up just like jogging.

The key to getting cardiovascular benefits from resistance training is high intensity work periods and short rest periods, so your heart rate remains elevated.

You can build muscle, increase your metabolism, and get the cardiovascular benefits all from one workout.

Resistance training is the best way to increase your metabolism so that your body is constantly burning calories.

You don't get this same benefit from jogging, walking, or running. In fact, lifting weights can turn up your metabolism so high that you can burn calories up to 48 hours after an intense session. Not true for the pure cardio sessions.

So, if you're looking to lose weight and melt off body fat, make sure you're lifting weights!

Don't be afraid you're going to get big bulky muscles by lifting weights because this is simply not true.

Women don't have enough testosterone to develop big bulky muscles. And as long as your caloric intake doesn't exceed the number of calories you burn daily, you won't get bigger.

12 Great Strength Training Exercises for Weight Loss

Here are some great strength training exercises.

1. Push-ups
2. Chest press
3. Squats
4. Reverse lunges
5. Seated row
6. Pull downs
7. Dips
8. Bicep curls
9. Planks
10. Shoulder press
11. Hip extensions
12. Crunches

These exercises work great because they are compound movements—meaning they work multiple muscle groups for one movement.

You will build more muscle, burn more calories, and lose more weight with these exercises compared to others.

The key to getting results with lifting weights is to do repetitions until failure—until you can't do any more.

Set a goal of performing an exercise for 10-15 repetitions. If you can go beyond 15, the weight or resistance you're using is too light/easy.

After you complete your set of 10-15 reps, wait 30 seconds to one minute depending on the shape you're in, and repeat the same exercise before moving on to the next.

Make sure you complete at least one exercise for each major muscle group; legs, chest, upper back, and midsection.

Also, make sure you follow a push pull sequence. Start with a pushing exercise like a push up, and then follow this by a pulling exercise like a pull down.

The Simplest, Quickest, and Most Effective Workout

Here's an example workout.

1. Chest press: 10 – 15 repetitions X 2
2. Seated row: 10 – 15 reps. X 2
3. Squats: 15 – 20 reps X 2
4. Hip extensions: 15 reps X 2
5. Plank: 30 – 60 seconds X 2
6. Shoulder press: 10 – 15 reps X 2
7. Bicep curls: 10 – 15 reps X 2
8. Dips: 10 – 15 reps X 2

This is a complete total body workout. Wait no longer than 60 seconds in between sets and exercises. Once you're in good shape cut your rest periods down to 30 seconds.

Great Exercises for Stress Relief

Resistance training and cardiovascular workouts can be stressful on the body, but as long as you follow the suggestions on time your body will recover and benefit from the workouts.

It's OK to be sore from workouts—muscle soreness usually peaks 48 hours after an intense session.

Soreness is a reflection of the effort you put into the workout. The first couple of weeks after starting a program are usually the most sensitive. After two weeks, your body will adapt and the soreness is minimal.

Other great forms of exercise to add to your routine especially for someone with hypothyroidism, include meditation, breathing exercises, stretching, and walking. Adding a couple sessions of meditation into your weekly routine will benefit you tremendously.

Most stress is a result of outside circumstances some of which you can't control. You can relieve this stress with practice of meditation, breathing, and changing your mindset. Believe it or not, how you process your thoughts is an exercise well worth pursuing.

Your Weekly Workout Routine

The best time to exercise is first thing in the morning because no one is calling you at 6:00 am to get your attention. It feels great to get exercise out of the way and it will give you energy the rest of the day.

Another reason is because this is a time when cortisol levels are naturally peaking and it's a good time to put this stress hormone to work.

Here is an example of a good weekly workout routine.

Monday—Lift weights

Tuesday—Cardio

Wednesday—Walk

Thursday—Lift weights

Friday—Cardio

Saturday—Meditate

Sunday—Stretch

I added the cardio sessions purely for variety. You can mix and match any of these workouts—just be sure you don't do two resistance workouts back to back because your body needs 48 to repair your muscles.

Don't be afraid to mix it up and try new exercises, use a variable number of repetitions and sets with higher and lower weights.

This will keep your body from adapting to your routine, which means you will always be burning more calories and building muscle.

There you have it...all the tools and ideas you'll need for a successful exercise program.

The key to successful weight loss with exercise is Frequency, followed by Intensity, Time, and Type.

Just remember the acronym for **FITT...Frequency, Intensity, Time, and Type.**

Be consistent with your program and you'll be successful.

Two Exercises Loaded with Health Benefits, Yet No One Does Them

There are two forms of exercise that are loaded with health benefits, yet you see no one doing them in a gym or even talking about them.

Do you remember the infomercials with a person jumping up and down on a mini trampoline?

It's called rebounding—and it has a ton of health benefits from helping your lymphatic system to increasing circulation to internal organs and increasing cellular respiration.

It sounds pretty technical, but all you have to know is that it can help your body function at a higher level; and when your body is working more efficiently, it will help you lose weight and ward off disease.

Another exercise is called total body vibration. It requires you to have access to a particular machine, but my guess is there's probably one in your town.

One machine that got a lot of press is called the Powerplate, but there are similar models, like the one I use with my patients called the Noblerex K 1.

They can be expensive, so I suggest you find one near you and pay per session instead of buying one.

Total body vibration has been used with professional athletes, celebrities, and Olympic athletes. It was originally designed to help astronauts increase bone density and muscle mass after long space missions.

Researchers also discovered this machine helps with weight loss, reduces cortisol, increases human growth hormone, and it gets results in just ten minutes!

So, if you can get access to this type of machine, use it!

The Most Important Exercise of All...

The only area of exercise that wasn't covered that is tremendously helpful in achieving your goals is the power of positive thinking and goal setting.

There are a number of books written on this subject, and it is well worth the time and investment to educate yourself on goal setting and how your subconscious mind works.

One of the major reasons people fail to achieve what they set out to accomplish is the fact that they have the wrong mindset.

Goal setting can be as simple as carrying a card with you that has your goals written on it. You can look at this card throughout the day to give yourself a reminder of why you're doing what you're doing.

It also helps to use visual imagery.

For example, think what you desire and picture yourself already in possession of it. Whether it's being thin, rich, or successful. It's as easy as picturing yourself already thin, rich, or successful.

However, the one thing that you must attach to the mental images is emotion!

Think about how you would feel if you could accomplish this...get excited about it!

Emotion is what gets you going and keeps you going.

Don't neglect this simple, yet powerful practice of controlling your mindset. It is the most powerful exercise there is.

Chapter 11

How to Find the Right Doctor for Your Thyroid Problem

There's no one that knows your body better than you and it can get very frustrating when you know there's something wrong with your health, yet your doctor tells you—you're fine.

This is a problem that is heard way too often by many patients, especially those with hypothyroidism.

<u>So, how can your blood test results come back normal and you still feel sick?</u>

Unfortunately, way too many doctors base their medical decisions purely upon test results, instead of listening to their patients and their symptoms.

However, there are doctors that will listen to you and believe you when you say there is something wrong.

Unfortunately, you may have to do some digging around to find the right doctor, and I'm going to help you find one that will get to the bottom of your problem.

Why Blood Tests Don't Always Work

The U.S. is the best place to live in the whole world, but it does have some drawbacks to living here and one drawback is the American medical model.

Don't get me wrong, the U.S. has the most sophisticated medical treatments available and the technology is far more advanced than anywhere else in the world, which I am thankful for.

But in my opinion, the medical model is based on diagnosing and treating disease. It's not one that focuses on optimizing health or catching health problems before they happen.

The U.S. has the most advanced medicine in the world, yet it has some of the sickest people in the world, and there are conditions that exist here and no place else.

Agriculture, the fast food industry, big drug companies, insurance companies, and lifestyle are partially to blame for all of this, but so is the sick-care system that is supported.

It's not your doctor's fault that he may misunderstand your symptoms for those of a healthy person; it's the system he was taught in medical school and it hasn't changed.

Most doctors run a blood test, and if your numbers are within the normal range—you're fine black and white, and that's how the insurance companies see it as well.

The problem with blood tests is that they're designed to identify SICK people, and the reference ranges used were based solely from people who are really sick.

<u>But what if you have some symptoms, and you're not really sick yet?</u>

Unfortunately, if you don't have numbers that represent a sick person, yet you still have symptoms, you will fall between the cracks and get lost in the medical system.

This is scenario # 1.

<u>You know you have a problem, your doctor thinks you may have a problem, but your numbers say you're fine. So, out the door you go, frustrated, sick, and hopefully onto a look for another doctor that will listen to you.</u>

Let's look at scenario # 2, which is more common.

<u>You've been battling hypothyroidism for a while, it's been diagnosed correctly, and you're being medicated for your problem—so everything is fine, right?</u>

Wrong.

You know you're not feeling right and you tell your doctor something's wrong, but he says you're fine according to your blood work.

Maybe there has been a change in your numbers, and maybe your doctor has made some adjustments with your medication, but you still don't feel well.

What's wrong here?

Well, maybe the medication you're taking is not the right medicine for you, so on to another prescription to see if it works.

You feel good for a while and then—bam, you feel the way you did months ago.

Now what?

<u>Is it possible that your problem can involve more than just your thyroid?</u>

You betcha...

Maybe you don't have a thyroid problem after all and it's your immune system going haywire and it's attacking your thyroid like it does with Hashimoto's thyroiditis.

By the way, Hashimoto's is the number one form of hypothyroidism in the US.

Do you try another doctor? Do you try another medication? Or maybe your doctor tells you that this is something you might have to live with.

I don't know about you, but if a doctor told me that I would have to deal with something the rest of my life—and I felt sick, you better believe I would look for some answers.

Unfortunately, the above scenarios are played out every day for people with hypothyroidism and many other conditions.

Do You Have the Right Tests?

One of the problems is that you may need another doctor, or it could be that the guidelines your doctor is using to evaluate your condition are not the most accurate.

The reference guidelines for test results that are commonly used are based upon results for those who are really sick with disease. This type of testing guideline is what's referred to as a <u>pathological range.</u>

This is the reference that most doctors and labs use.

In other words, the only people who are put into this category are those who are seriously ill and have a pathological condition.

But what if you are just on the edge of being sick, or you have a condition like hypothyroidism and your numbers say you're fine because you're being medicated, yet you still don't feel right?

Now what?

<u>This is where millions of Americans who are not feeling well fall in between the cracks and get lost in the American medical model.</u>

Is there a solution? Yes!

One solution is to find a doctor that can diagnose your condition correctly and treat your immune system naturally.

I will show you how and where to look for such a physician.

The other important factor in trying to figure out if you have hypothyroidism or an immune problem like Hashimoto's is to make sure your doctor is using a functional reference guide for blood test results and not a pathological reference guide.

A <u>functional reference guide</u> allows doctors and labs to identify patients that are subclinical or may not have symptoms but test results show there is a problem.

Or you may have mild symptoms, or your test results may be just a little off. This range is important, so patients can be identified earlier than later.

The important thing is to get your doctor to perform all the right tests, use the right reference guide and take your clinical symptoms into account.

You now know the difference between pathological and functional reference ranges for blood tests and I am going to tell you exactly what tests are needed and what your numbers should look like.

The Only Tests You'll Need for Hypothyroidism

Listed below you'll find 11 tests that should be run if there is a hunch that you may have hypothyroidism. Because there are different causes and treatments for hypothyroidism, you should get all these tests performed.

Test	Function Range
TSH - thyroid stimulating hormone	1.8–3.0 mlu/l
TT4—total thyroxine	6-12 ug/dl
TT3—triiodothyronine	100-180 ng/dl
Free T4	1.0-1.5 ng/dl
Free thyroxine index	1.2-4.9 mg/dl
Free T3	3.0-4.0 pg/ml
T3 uptake	28-38 md/dl
Reverse T3	25-30 ng/dl
Thyroid binding globulin	18-27 ug/dl
Thyroid perioxidase antibody	above lab range
Antithyroglobulin antibody	above lab range

Questions to Ask to Find the Right Physician

Trying to find a physician that knows how to diagnose and treat a condition that has many causes and variable symptoms is like trying to find a needle in a haystack.

But if you arm yourself with the right questions before your first visit— your chances will be better than most.

Put yourself in the doctor's shoes for just a moment...

In walks a patient complaining with symptoms of fatigue, weight-gain, depression, dry skin, constipation, and low libido. Without taking a history of your health or performing any test, the symptoms you described could be any number of conditions.

In fact, if you were to talk to 10 random females age 35-50, you could be sure that 3 or 4 of them would tell you that they suffer from more than one of those symptoms.

<u>Hypothyroidism has many symptoms, many causes, and blood test results can vary for the same person month to month, especially if they have Hashimoto's.</u>

So, you can see how this may be a daunting task for any physician who sees multiple cases like this every day and many have different outcomes.

Not only will you be helping yourself to find the right physician by asking the right questions, but you will be helping the doctor in the process.

And this may be easier than you think.

The first thing to do is to ask a friend or relative if they know a local endocrinologist.

Chances are you'll get a couple of recommendations.

Try to get as much information from your friend about the doctor as possible, because in most cases it's impossible to get a doctor on the phone.

If your friend doesn't know the answers to your questions, try to get answers from the physician's website if they have one. If they don't have a website, call their office and ask to speak with the doctor directly.

Your last resort is to talk with someone on their staff such as a nurse.

Most docs have an email address, so ask if you can send them an email with some questions—or try a text message.

<u>This is your health we're talking about, so be persistent about perusing the answers to these questions until you feel confident you have the right doctor.</u>

You need to do your homework; it will save you time, energy, and money.

Here are 10 questions to ask:

1. What test(s) do you run to determine hypothyroidism?
   If the doctor just runs a TSH test, move on and keep looking for a doctor.

2. **Do you use a pathological or functional reference range to compare test results?**
   Make sure the doctor uses a functional reference guide.

3. **How often will you test my thyroid if I need medication?**
   If the doctor doesn't initially run a monthly thyroid panel, move on.

4. **What are my treatment options if I have hypothyroidism?**
   Some people will respond better to some medications than others, so ask about medication options. If there is only one type of medication they use—look for another doctor.

5. **How many types of thyroid problems are there?**
   If he or she mentions there is only hyperthyroidism or hypothyroidism—move on.

6. **Can you tell me what caused my hypothyroidism?**
   If the doctor tells you there is no way of knowing what caused your hypothyroidism—run! If they can't figure out what caused it, they will not be able to treat it successfully.

7. **Will you run an antibody test on my thyroid?**
   If your doctor won't run a thyroid antibody test, find another doctor because most forms of hypothyroidism are Hashimoto's and this is determined through a thyroid antibody test.

8. **How do you treat the immune system?**
   The number one cause of hypothyroidism is Hashimoto's, which is an immune system problem. If you have Hashimoto's, you will need to address your immune system. If your doctor doesn't do this, you will need to find one that will.

9. **Will eating a certain way make my condition better or worse?**
   If the doctor suggests your diet has nothing to do with how you feel, find a good nutritionist.

10. Can you tell me some success stories about your patients?
If they don't have much to say or they are not specific and mention names or reference,s chances are they might not have too much success with your condition.

Hire the Right Doctor

Think about this as an interview process—which it is. Pretend you're the boss and you're looking for an employee and that this hire will make or break your company.

The sad thing is, most people will go to see any doctor regardless of how good or bad they may be or without knowing much about this person and put their life in his/her hands.

Doctors are human beings; there are good ones and bad ones, and it's your responsibility to find out if they're the best and don't expect anything less.

Most people who own companies will go through rigorous interviews to find the best qualified person to work for them; but when it comes to their health, people can't be bothered to take the time to ask a few questions.

The best way to think about this process is if you have kids, pretend you're looking for a specialist for your child who has a rare life-threatening disease and you only have one shot to get it right.

Get it right the first time!

Conclusion

Hypothyroidism and its symptoms are due to environmental, hereditary, diet, and lifestyle factors. You cannot control your genetics, but you can control the lifestyle factors that transform a genetic predisposition into a symptomatic condition.

Once your hypothyroidism "switch" has been flipped on and you acknowledge you have it, there won't be one pill that can turn it off.

If you rely solely on the current medical system to cure your condition, you will lose your battle against the disease.

However, if you educate yourself and take control of your health by reducing your toxic exposure, eliminate food allergies/sensitivities, and support your immune system, you can dramatically reduce your symptoms or even eliminate them altogether.

Weight gain is just one symptom of hypothyroidism and is the result of a depressed metabolism.

Even though your thyroid is the master gland of metabolism, there are certain things that you can do to speed it up.

Things such as what you eat, when you eat, exercise, and reducing certain stressors on your body can have a huge impact on your metabolism.

Don't underestimate the power of supplements and exercise and how they can impact your health. Treat both as medicine and, when in doubt, consult with a specialist.

None of this information can take the place of being treated and examined by a licensed medical doctor.

Health professionals such as Chiropractors, Naprapaths, Naturopaths, Nutritionists, and Personal Trainers should be a strong consideration for your healthcare team in your battle against weight loss, hypothyroidism, or any other illness that you may encounter in life.

Remember, it's not one pill or potion that will keep you healthy, it's a well-rounded support program and team...and you're the leader.

Eat well and be well,

Dr. Kevin Dobrzynski DN

About the Author

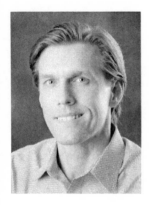

Dr. Kevin Dobrzynski DN attended The University of Rhode Island for his undergraduate studies, where he also competed in collegiate football and specialized in sports medicine.

He continued his education at The Chicago National College of Naprapathy, where he graduated with honors.

He is currently licensed in Illinois as a Doctor of Naprapathy.

Kevin is also a certified personal trainer through the National Academy of Sports Medicine and he is a Metabolic Typing Advisor through healthexcel.

Dr. Dobrzynski uses exercise prescription along with nutritional counseling and supplementation to create the backbone of his practice. He believes that exercise and correct nutrition play an essential role in preventing and rehabilitating the body of DISEASE.

"Combining alternative medicine with exercise creates a healthy option and balance to give you the freedom while staying in control of your own healthcare."

His love of nutrition and fitness and genuine concern for others drive his pursuit of excellence in his work, as well as his service to the community.

Kevin's goal is to expose as many people as possible to the best natural health resources so that others can stay in control of their own health. *Kevin has been practicing in the suburbs of Chicago for 10 years.* He is married to wife Amy and together they are raising two healthy children, Brook 5 and Dean 3.

FREE Membership

Claim Your FREE Membership and Bonuses... A $97 Value for Book Buyers Only! @ TheHypothyroidDiet.com/**Members**

Your membership will help you answer common questions; clear up any confusion, and most importantly, it will help you beat hypothyroidism.

With your membership you can...

- **Get insider information on supplements that work**
- Increase your likelihood of success
- **Get groundbreaking nutrition information**
- Listen to expert interviews
- **Get updated information on weight loss, depression, & fatigue**
- Receive special discount rates on products and services
- **Listen to FREE webinars, teleseminars, and more...**

You don't have to do this alone...join our community for support and get informed about new discoveries and hypothyroidism.

Use Your Cell Phone to Scan The Bar Code Below and Go Directly to TheHypothyroidDiet.com/**Members** Area Now for Your FREE Bonuses!

BUY A SHARE OF THE FUTURE IN YOUR COMMUNITY

These certificates make great holiday, graduation and birthday gifts that can be personalized with the recipient's name. The cost of one S.H.A.R.E. or one square foot is $54.17. The personalized certificate is suitable for framing and will state the number of shares purchased and the amount of each share, as well as the recipient's name. The home that you participate in "building" will last for many years and will continue to grow in value.

Here is a sample SHARE certificate:

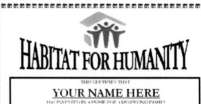

YES, I WOULD LIKE TO HELP!

I support the work that Habitat for Humanity does and I want to be part of the excitement! As a donor, I will receive periodic updates on your construction activities but, more importantly, I know my gift will help a family in our community realize the dream of homeownership. I would like to SHARE in your efforts against substandard housing in my community! (Please print below)

PLEASE SEND ME _____ SHARES at $54.17 EACH = $ $_____

In Honor Of: _____

Occasion: (Circle One) HOLIDAY BIRTHDAY ANNIVERSARY

OTHER: _____

Address of Recipient: _____

Gift From: _____ *Donor Address:* _____

Donor Email: _____

I AM ENCLOSING A CHECK FOR $ $_____ PAYABLE TO HABITAT FOR HUMANITY <u>OR</u> PLEASE CHARGE MY VISA OR MASTERCARD *(CIRCLE ONE)*

Card Number _____ Expiration Date: _____

Name as it appears on Credit Card _____ Charge Amount $ _____

Signature _____

Billing Address _____

Telephone # Day _____ Eve _____

PLEASE NOTE: Your contribution is tax-deductible to the fullest extent allowed by law.
Habitat for Humanity • P.O. Box 1443 • Newport News, VA 23601 • 757-596-5553
www.HelpHabitatforHumanity.org

CPSIA information can be obtained at www.ICGtesting.com
Printed in the USA
BVOW08s2230061113

335688BV00004B/73/P